Regina

DRUGS OF CHOICE FROM THE MEDICAL LETTER

Published by

The Medical Letter, Inc.
1000 Main Street
New Rochelle, New York 10801-7537

(ISSN 1065-6596)
The Medical Letter, Inc.
1000 Main Street
New Rochelle, New York 10801-7537

CONTENTS

DRUGS FOR STABLE ANGINA PECTORIS

Many nitrates, beta-blockers and calcium-channel blockers have now been approved by the US Food and Drug Administration for treatment of stable angina pectoris. The table beginning on page 9 lists the individual drugs, their dosage and their cost.

NITRATES — Nitrates are potent venous and arterial dilators. They decrease venous return and myocardial oxygen demand and increase collateral blood flow to ischemic areas (J Abrams, Arch Intern Med, 155:357, 1995). All nitrates can cause rapid development of tolerance, but a drug-free interval overnight can reverse the tolerance that develops during the day.

Nitroglycerin – Sublingual nitroglycerin is the drug of choice for an acute attack of angina. The therapeutic effect lasts for less than an hour, making it unsuitable for long-term prophylaxis, but in patients who have angina associated with physical activity, sublingual nitroglycerin taken five to ten minutes before the activity can prevent or delay an attack. A translingual spray is as effective as the sublingual tablets and has the same indications (Medical Letter, 28:59, 1986). Nitroglycerin is also available in an extended-release transmucosal tablet (Medical Letter, 29:39, 1987). The absorption of swallowed nitroglycerin is poor, and its effectiveness for long-term treatment has never been established.

Absorption of transdermal nitroglycerin from skin varies in different patients and at different sites of application. One to two inches of nitroglycerin ointment (2%) applied over an area of 36 square inches three or four times a day and removed for 10 to 12 hours during each 24-hour period is effective for short-term treatment of angina, but its long-term effectiveness has never been established. Continuous use of nitroglycerin patches causes rapid development of tolerance. Intermittent treatment with the patches — leaving them off for 10 to 12 hours overnight — prevents development of tolerance but may cause rebound nocturnal angina and decrease early-morning exercise capacity (Medical Letter, 31:65, 1989; Steering Committee, Am J Cardiol, 68:1263, 1991).

Isosorbide Dinitrate – Sublingual isosorbide dinitrate is slower in onset of action than sublingual nitroglycerin and less effective for treatment of acute angina. Its one-to-two-hour duration of action does make it suitable, however, for prevention of angina during physical exertion. Use of oral isosorbide dinitrate four times a day leads to tolerance, but taking it two or three times a day in the morning and afternoon can prevent tolerance (JO Parker et al, N Engl J Med, 316:1440, 1987). The long-term effectiveness of oral slow-release formulations of isosorbide dinitrate has not been established. In one trial, a 40-mg sustained-release formulation t.i.d. was not superior to placebo (RG Friedman et al, J Invasive Cardiol, 4:319, 1992).

Isosorbide-5-Mononitrate – Isosorbide-5-mononitrate is the major active metabolite of isosorbide dinitrate. Unlike the dinitrate, it is nearly 100% bioavailable and has no active metabolites. Twice-daily treatment in the morning and afternoon does not produce tolerance or rebound nocturnal angina (JO Parker et al, Am J Cardiol, 72:871, 1993; U Thadani et al, Ann Intern Med, 120:353, 1994). A controlled-release form of isosorbide mononitrate *(Imdur)* was recently marketed in the USA; once-daily doses appear to be effective without producing tolerance (SG Chrysant et al, Am J Cardiol, 72:1249, 1993; Medical Letter, 36:13, 1994).

Adverse Effects – Nitrates are generally well tolerated. The most common adverse effect is headache, which occurs in 30% to 60% of patients taking long-acting nitrates. Occasionally, headaches may be severe and associated with nausea and prostration. Some patients develop symptomatic postural hypotension, and syncope can occur.

BETA-ADRENERGIC BLOCKERS — Beta-blockers decrease myocardial oxygen demand by decreasing heart rate, contractility, and systolic blood pressure during exercise. By slowing the heart rate, they prolong diastolic filling, making more time available for coronary blood flow. Of all the available antianginal drugs, beta-blockers without intrinsic sympathomimetic activity (all except acebutolol, carteolol, penbutolol and pindolol) are the most effective in decreasing myocardial ischemia (AA Quyyumi et al, Br Heart J, 57:505, 1987; PH Stone et al, Circulation, 82:1962, 1990). In post-infarction patients, controlled trials have shown that a beta-blocker can decrease the risk of another myocardial infarction and death (S Yusof et al, JAMA, 260:2088, 1988).

Adverse Effects – In general, beta-blockers are well tolerated. Because of their negative inotropic effects, they can precipitate or aggravate heart failure. Symptomatic bradycardia, hypotension, fatigue, depression, cold extremities, impotence, constipation and vivid dreams can occur. In diabetic patients who develop hypoglycemia, beta-blockers can mask some of the symptoms and delay recovery. Even cardioselective beta-blockers can produce severe bronchospasm in patients with asthma or other reactive airway disease. Sudden withdrawal of a beta-blocker can exacerbate angina or lead to a myocardial infarction; gradual withdrawal over several days is recommended. Beta-blockers are contraindicated in patients with Raynaud's phenomenon and those with pain at rest due to peripheral vascular disease. Beta-blockers used concurrently with verapamil or diltiazem may have marked negative inotropic effects and may cause bradycardia and occasionally high-grade AV block.

CALCIUM-CHANNEL BLOCKERS — Calcium-channel blockers decrease myocardial oxygen demand and increase coronary blood flow. Verapamil and diltiazem also decrease exercise-induced increases in heart rate (D Acanfora et al, G Ital Cardiol, 23:451, 1993; U Thadani et al, Am J Cardiol, 74:9, 1994). All of the calcium-channel blockers currently available in the USA except diltiazem, verapamil and bepridil are dihydropyridines.

Choice of Drugs – A calcium-channel blocker is the drug of choice for patients with both angina and hypertension who cannot take a beta-blocker. In patients with angina who also have episodes of supraventricular tachycardia, verapamil or diltiazem is effective for both, but the dihydropyridines are not and can aggravate the arrhythmia. Therapeutic doses of amlodipine generally do not have a negative inotropic effect (D Murdoch and RC Heel, Drugs, 41:478, 1991), and the drug has been used in small numbers of patients with depressed left ventricular function without aggravating heart failure (Medical Letter, 34:99, 1992), but adequate controlled trials in patients with heart failure are not available. Bepridil alone or added to other drugs may be more effective than other calcium-channel blockers for treatment of refractory angina (BN Singh, Am J Cardiol, 68:306, 1991; Medical Letter, 33:53, 1991), but it can cause serious adverse effects.

Adverse Effects – In general, calcium-channel blockers are well tolerated; they can cause vasodilator effects such as headache, flushing and dizziness. They can also precipitate heart failure in patients with compromised left ventricular function, particularly if verapamil or diltiazem is used with a beta-blocker. Verapamil and diltiazem are more likely to suppress cardiac contractility and slow cardiac conduction; the dihydropyridines are more potent vasodilators. Peripheral edema secondary to vasodilation occurs more often with dihydropyridines than with diltiazem or verapamil. Constipation is often a problem with verapamil, especially in the elderly. Bradycardia or high-degree AV block may develop with diltiazem or verapamil, especially if they are used with a beta-blocker. The dihydropyridines can induce angina due to reflex tachycardia secondary to vasodilatation; these effects are rare, however, with amlodipine or slow-release formulations of nifedipine. Concurrent use of a beta-blocker can decrease both the tachycardia and the angina. Bepridil prolongs the QT interval and can cause torsades de pointes, a serious ventricular arrhythmia, especially in patients with hypokalemia (P Coumel, Am J Cardiol, 69:75D, 1992).

CONCLUSION — Nitrates, beta-blockers and calcium-channel blockers are all effective for treatment of angina pectoris. When the response to one type of drug is inadequate, a second and sometimes a third may be added. Only beta-blockers after myocardial infarction have been shown to decrease mortality.

DRUGS FOR STABLE ANGINA PECTORIS

Drug	Dosage	Cost*
NITRATES		
Nitroglycerin		
sublingual tablets – *Nitrostat* (Parke-Davis)	0.3 to 0.6 mg PRN (up to 3 tablets)	$ 6.18[1]
translingual spray – *Nitrolingual* (Rhône-Poulenc Rorer)	0.4 mg/spray (up to 3 sprays)	23.83[2]
transmucosal tablets – *Nitrogard* (Forest)	1 to 3 mg q5h 3x/day	36.07
oral extended-release	2.5 to 6.5 bid to qid	
average generic price (capsules)		4.46
Nitroglyn E-R (Kenwood)		4.78
Nitrong (Rhône-Poulenc Rorer)		18.34
ointment – 2%	1" to 2" q4h for 12 to 14 hours/day	
average generic price		9.85[3]
Nitro-Bid (Marion-Merrell Dow)		6.50[3]
transdermal patches[4]	one patch 12 to 14 hours/day	
average generic price		41.95[5]
Deponit (Schwarz)		47.15[5]
Minitran (3M)		41.28[5]
Nitrodisc (Searle)		48.17[5]
Nitro-Dur (Key)		44.57[5]
Transderm-Nitro (Ciba)		52.08[5]
Isosorbide Dinitrate		
sublingual tablets – immediate release	2.5 to 10 mg q2-3h	
average generic price		4.13[1]
Isordil (Wyeth-Ayerst)		22.91[1]
Sorbitrate (Zeneca)		18.62[1]

(continued)

* Cost to the pharmacist for 30 days' treatment (unless otherwise noted) with lowest recommended dose based on wholesale price (AWP) listings in *Drug Topics Red Book* 1995 and May *Update*.

1. Cost of one bottle of 100 tablets.
2. One canister (14.49 grams) containing 200 0.4-mg metered doses.
3. Cost of one 60-gram tube. One inch of ointment contains 15 mg of nitroglycerin.
4. Nitroglycerin patches are available in sizes ranging from 0.1 mg/hour to 0.8 mg/hour (formerly 2.5 mg to 20 mg/24 hours).
5. Cost of 30 patches delivering 0.4 mg/hour.

Drug	Dosage	Cost*
Isosorbide Dinitrate *(continued)*		
oral tablets	30 mg bid or 20 mg tid in morning and afternoon	
average generic price		$ 2.92
Isordil Titradose		29.95
Sorbitrate		24.36
extended-release tablets and capsules	40 to 80 mg once daily to tid	
average generic price		2.38
Isordil Tembids		15.75
Dilatrate SR (Reed & Carnrick)		14.48
Isosorbide-5-Mononitrate		
immediate release	20 mg in morning and afternoon, 7 hours apart	
ISMO (Wyeth-Ayerst)		39.49
Monoket (Schwarz)		31.59
extended-release	60 to 120 mg once daily	
Imdur (Schering/Key)		23.93
BETA-BLOCKERS		
Atenolol	50 to 100 mg once daily	
average generic price		19.53
Tenormin (Zeneca)		27.06
Metoprolol	50 to 200 mg bid	
average generic price		27.10
Lopressor (Geigy)		31.23
Nadolol	40 to 80 mg once daily	
average generic price		25.91
Corgard (Bristol)		33.35
Propranolol		
immediate release	80 to 320 mg divided bid, tid, or qid	
average generic price		5.91
Inderal (Wyeth-Ayerst)		34.19
extended release	80 to 160 mg once daily	
average generic price		23.05
Inderal LA		26.91
CALCIUM-CHANNEL BLOCKERS		
Dihydropyridines		
Amlodipine – *Norvasc* (Pfizer)	5 to 10 mg once daily	35.36
Nicardipine – *Cardene* (Syntex)	20 to 40 mg tid	36.64
Nifedipine		
immediate release	10 to 30 mg tid or qid	
average generic price		38.80
Adalat (Miles)		41.86
Procardia (Pfizer)		54.52

Drug	Dosage	Cost*
Calcium-Channel Blockers *(continued)*		
Nifedipine		
extended-release		
Procardia XL	30 to 90 mg once daily	$ 36.96
Other Classes		
Diltiazem		
immediate release	30 to 120 mg tid or qid	
average generic price		32.81
Cardizem (Marion-Merrell Dow)		39.15
extended-release		
Cardizem CD	120 to 480 mg once daily	31.32
Verapamil	80 to 120 mg tid or qid	
average generic price		20.48
Calan (Searle)		42.95
Isoptin (Knoll)		39.81
Bepridil – *Vascor* (McNeil)	200 to 400 mg once daily	70.10

* Cost to the pharmacist for 30 days' treatment (unless otherwise noted) with lowest recommended dose based on wholesale price (AWP) listings in *Drug Topics Red Book* 1995 and May *Update*.

DRUGS FOR RHEUMATOID ARTHRITIS

Many different drugs are now used to treat rheumatoid arthritis. Aspirin and the other nonsteroidal anti-inflammatory drugs (NSAIDs) listed in the table on page 20 have analgesic and anti-inflammatory effects, and they are relatively safe. The second-line drugs listed on page 22 have no immediate analgesic effects, but they can control symptoms and may delay progression of the disease. NSAIDs usually are taken concurrently with the slower acting second-line drugs, which, with the exception of methotrexate, may take months to produce a therapeutic response (JM Cash and JH Klippel, N Engl J Med, 330:1368, 1994).

NSAIDS — Aspirin in high doses is as effective as any other NSAID and much less expensive, but many patients cannot tolerate its gastrointestinal toxicity. No NSAID is consistently more effective than any other, but some patients who do not respond to or tolerate one may respond to or tolerate another.

Adverse Effects – It is not clear whether an equally effective dose of any NSAID is safer than any other. All NSAIDs can cause dyspepsia and gastrointestinal toxicity, including gastric and duodenal ulceration and perforation, with or without warning symptoms, especially in elderly patients treated chronically with these agents. All NSAIDs except the nonacetylated salicylates can interfere with platelet function and prolong bleeding time. Except with aspirin, this effect is reversible when the drug is cleared, but the combination of gastrointestinal irritation and prolonged bleeding time can cause serious gastrointestinal hemorrhage, especially in elderly patients. Some studies have found that ibuprofen (*Motrin*, and others) and naproxen (*Naprosyn*, and others) have a lower risk of serious gastrointestinal complications than other NSAIDs (LA Garcia Rodriguez and H Jick, Lancet, 343:769, 1994). Nabumetone *(Relafen)* may cause less gastric irritation than other NSAIDs (Medical Letter, 34:38, 1992). Meclofenamate (*Meclomen*, and others) may cause a high incidence of diarrhea, which is sometimes severe. Piroxicam (*Feldene*, and others), which has a longer half-life and may cause a higher incidence of gastrointestinal bleeding than other NSAIDs, should be avoided in elderly patients. Misoprostol *(Cytotec)*, a prostaglandin analog, can prevent gastric ulceration caused by NSAIDs (DY Graham et al, Ann Intern Med, 119:257, 1993).

NSAIDs decrease renal blood flow, cause fluid retention and may cause renal failure in some patients, particularly the elderly (D Schlondorff, Kidney Int, 44:643, 1993). Diminished renal function and decreased effective intravascular volume due to diuretic therapy, cirrhosis or congestive heart failure may increase the risk of renal toxicity. Renal papillary necrosis, interstitial nephritis and the nephrotic syndrome occur rarely.

All NSAIDs can cause central-nervous-system (CNS) effects such as dizziness, anxiety, drowsiness and confusion; these symptoms may occur initially and disappear with further use. Indomethacin (*Indocin*, and others) may cause more severe CNS adverse effects than other NSAIDs; depression, disorientation and, especially, severe headache occur frequently with higher doses. Tinnitus has been associated particularly with high doses of salicylates. Aseptic meningitis has occurred rarely in patients with lupus erythematosus or other connective tissue diseases who were taking ibuprofen, tolmetin (*Tolectin*, and others) or sulindac (*Clinoril*, and others) and has been reported with ibuprofen and naproxen in patients without any connective tissue disease.

NSAIDs frequently cause small increases in hepatic enzyme activity, but life-threatening hepatic toxicity is rare (LA Garcia Rodriguez et al, Arch Intern Med, 154:311, 1994). Pancreatitis has been reported. NSAIDs rarely cause blood dyscrasias; aplastic anemia has been reported with ibuprofen, fenoprofen (*Nalfon*, and others), naproxen, indomethacin, tolmetin and piroxicam. Asthmatic patients sensitive to aspirin could develop severe bronchospasm and anaphylactoid reactions with any NSAID. Various types of dermatological toxicity have been reported with NSAIDs, including toxic epidermal necrolysis. NSAIDs may interact with many other drugs; they may, for example, decrease the effectiveness of diuretics, beta-blockers, ACE inhibitors and some other antihypertensive drugs (*The Medical Letter Handbook of Adverse Drug Interactions*, 1995, page 208).

SECOND-LINE DRUGS — Failure to achieve or maintain an adequate response with an NSAID alone calls for addition of a second-line drug – often hydroxychloroquine for mild rheumatoid arthritis or methotrexate if the disease is more severe. Many clinicians now do not wait for an NSAID response but begin therapy with a second-line drug at the time of diagnosis. All second-line drugs require regular monitoring for adverse effects.

HYDROXYCHLOROQUINE *(Plaquenil)* — The antimalarial hydroxychloroquine in doses of 200 mg to 400 mg daily is frequently effective for rheumatoid arthritis and is usually well tolerated (ED Harris, Ann Intern Med, 119:1146, 1993; HERA Study Group, Am J Med, 98:156, 1995). Nausea and epigastric pain can occur, but serious adverse effects are rare. Retinal damage has occurred, but can generally be avoided if vision is monitored (visual fields, color vision) at six to twelve month intervals and the drug is discontinued promptly when signs of retinal toxicity first appear.

METHOTREXATE (*Rheumatrex*, and others) — Oral methotrexate in low dosage decreases the symptoms of rheumatoid arthritis, and some rheumatologists now consider it a first-line drug (ME Weinblatt, N Engl J Med, 332:330, 1995). Medical Letter consultants recommend starting with 5 to 7.5 mg once a week, which can be increased gradually to 15 to 20 mg per week. Taking the drug weekly in two doses 12 hours apart has not been more effective or safer than a single weekly dose. The antirheumatic effect of low-dosage once-weekly methotrexate is often apparent within four to six weeks of treatment. For patients who have gastrointestinal effects or lose benefit over time with oral methotrexate, giving the same dose intramuscularly once weekly may be helpful. Some clinicians do not prescribe methotrexate for patients with a serum creatinine concentration higher than 2 mg/dL.

Adverse Effects — In low dosage, methotrexate is often well tolerated, but it commonly causes anorexia, nausea, vomiting, abdominal cramps and increased hepatic enzyme activity, and rarely bone marrow suppression, pulmonary toxicity and hepatic fibrosis. Hypersensitivity pneumonitis, frequently severe, occurs in 1% to 4% of rheumatoid arthritis patients taking methotrexate. The drug is immunosuppressive; infections such as herpes zoster and *Pneumocystis carinii* have been reported to be more common in patients taking methotrexate for rheumatoid arthritis (MAS Antonelli et al, Am J Med, 90:295, 1991; A Wollner et al, Thorax, 46:205, 1991). Lymphomas associated with Epstein-Barr virus have occurred during methotrexate therapy for rheumatoid arthritis and regressed completely after the drug was stopped (OW Kamel et al, N Engl J Med, 328:1317, 1993). Trimethoprim/sulfamethoxazole (*Bactrim*, and others) and possibly sulfasalazine (*Azulfidine*, and others) may increase bone marrow suppression due to methotrexate (H Groenendal and FHJ Rampen, Clin Exp Dermatol, 15:358, 1990).

Patients taking methotrexate require close monitoring for hepatic toxicity (JM Kremer et al, Arthritis Rheum, 37:316, 1994). Leucovorin, 2.5 to 5 mg, given 24 hours after the methotrexate dose may decrease the severity of nausea, mucosal ulceration and hepatic toxicity (JB Shiroky et al, Arthritis Rheum, 36:795, 1993). Some clinicians recommend folic acid to avoid folate depletion (SL Morgan et al, Ann Intern Med, 121:833, 1994). Methotrexate is teratogenic and should not be given to women who are or may become pregnant. It is also an abortifacient and can impair fertility in both men and women. In elderly patients or others with decreased renal function, concurrent use of an NSAID may increase serum concentrations and the toxicity of methotrexate (*Medical Letter Handbook of Adverse Drug Interactions*, 1995, page 182).

GOLD — Gold salts have been used for many years for treatment of severe rheumatoid arthritis. Recently, some clinicians have questioned their effectiveness (WV Epstein, Semin Arthritis Rheum, 23:32, 1994), but one meta-analysis placed them among the more effective of the second-line drugs (DT Felson, Arthritis Rheum, 35:1117, 1992). Gold sodium thiomalate *(Myochrysine)* and aurothioglucose *(Solganal)* are the two injectable preparations available in the USA. An oral preparation, auranofin *(Ridaura)*, is also available; it is generally less effective than injectable gold.

Dosage – The usual dosage of injectable gold includes a test dose of 10 mg, followed one week later by 25 mg once a week for two weeks, and then 50 mg weekly for up to 20 weeks. If a response occurs, treatment intervals may increase to every two weeks, then every three weeks, and then monthly. Response usually occurs within three to six months after starting treatment. Patients who respond should remain at least on monthly therapy; discontinuing maintenance gold therapy often results in recurrence of arthritis that may not remit when gold is re-instituted.

The dosage of auranofin is 3 mg twice a day or 6 mg once daily. If the disease does not respond, dosage may be increased to 3 mg t.i.d. if tolerated. If the response is still unsatisfactory, the drug should be discontinued.

Adverse Effects – Many patients have to discontinue injectable gold because of adverse effects, particularly stomatitis, rash, proteinuria, leukopenia and thrombocytopenia. Some clinicians obtain a complete blood count and urinalysis before each injection or every other injection to detect drug-related cytopenia or proteinuria. Pruritic rash and stomatitis sometimes resolve if therapy is withheld for a few weeks and then re-started cautiously at a lower dose. Enterocolitis and aplastic anemia are rare but potentially fatal adverse effects. Interstitial pneumonitis is another rare but serious adverse effect. Gold thiomalate uncommonly causes a "nitritoid" reaction characterized by flushing, weakness, nausea and dizziness within 30 minutes of injection. These reactions, which are usually mild, rarely occur with aurothioglucose. Oral gold causes less mucocutaneous, bone marrow and renal toxicity than injectable gold, but more diarrhea and other gastrointestinal reactions. Gold therapy is generally not recommended during pregnancy or lactation.

SULFASALAZINE (*Azulfidine,* and others) — Although not approved for such use by the US Food and Drug Administration (FDA), sulfasalazine in recent years has become increasingly popular as a treatment for rheumatoid arthritis. A meta-analysis of short-term clinical trials found sulfasalazine to be among the most effective second-line drugs (DT Felson et al, Arthritis Rheum,

35:1117, 1992). Its toxicity, however, may be greater than that of methotrexate or hydroxychloroquine. Two small studies have suggested that sulfasalazine may slow the progression of joint damage (DM Van der Heijde et al, Lancet, 335:539, 1990; P Hannonen et al, Arthritis Rheum, 36:1501, 1993).

Adverse Effects — Nausea, anorexia, and rash are fairly common with sulfasalazine, but serious reactions such as hepatitis and blood dyscrasias are rare. Sperm counts may decrease, but return to normal after withdrawal of the drug. Enteric-coated sulfasalazine decreases gastrointestinal toxicity.

PENICILLAMINE ***(Depen, Cuprimine)*** — Penicillamine can be effective in patients with refractory rheumatoid arthritis and may delay progression of erosions. The manufacturer recommends beginning with 125 or 250 mg once a day and slowly (at one- to three-month intervals) increasing by 125- or 250-mg increments up to 1000 and rarely to 1500 mg per day. Penicillamine should be taken between meals because food decreases its absorption.

Adverse Effects — The most common adverse effects of penicillamine are similar to those of parenteral gold – pruritic rash, proteinuria, aphthous ulcers, leukopenia and thrombocytopenia (HG Taylor and A Samanta, Drug Safety, 7:46, 1992). Anorexia, nausea and transient decreased or altered taste (dysgeusia) are also relatively common adverse effects. Rarely, pemphigus, myasthenia gravis, Goodpasture's syndrome, fever, lupus-like illness, polymyositis, dermatomyositis, cholestatic hepatitis, severe bone marrow depression and bronchiolitis can occur. Penicillamine is teratogenic and should not be used during pregnancy.

AZATHIOPRINE ***(Imuran)*** — Azathioprine, a purine analog immunosuppressive drug, given in a dosage of 1 to 2.5 mg/kg/day can be effective for refractory rheumatoid arthritis, but some patients cannot tolerate it.

Adverse Effects — Nausea, vomiting, abdominal pain, hepatitis and reversible bone marrow depression can occur with azathioprine. Severe toxicity is uncommon with the dosage used for rheumatoid arthritis, but an increased risk of lymphoma has been reported. Concurrent use of allopurinol (*Zyloprim*, and others) can increase the toxicity of azathioprine (*Medical Letter Handbook of Adverse Drug Interactions*, 1995, page 63). Azathioprine is not recommended for use during pregnancy.

CORTICOSTEROIDS — Use of corticosteroids in rheumatoid arthritis is controversial (MH Weisman, Rheum Dis Clin North Am, 19:189, 1993). Many patients who have an inadequate response or are intolerant to second-line agents benefit from 5 to 10 mg of prednisone per day or less. Low-dose prednisone may be especially useful in elderly patients as an alternative to the risks and inconvenience associated with second-line drugs and in younger patients to control active disease temporarily until second-line drugs with a slower onset of action can provide sufficient control. Corticosteroids in higher doses may be required to control severe systemic manifestations of rheumatoid arthritis, such as pericarditis or vasculitis. Intra-articular injection of a corticosteroid often can relieve an acutely inflamed rheumatoid joint with fewer systemic consequences than oral or intravenous preparations.

Adverse Effects — The adverse effects of systemic corticosteroids include osteoporosis, cataracts, poor wound healing, gastric ulcers, gastrointestinal bleeding, hyperglycemia, hypertension, adrenal suppression and increased risk of infection (KG Saag et al, Am J Med, 96:115, 1994). Even short-term use in low doses can cause bone loss (RFJM Laan et al, Ann Intern Med, 119:963, 1993).

CAPSAICIN (*Zostrix-HP,* and others) — An alkaloid found in hot peppers, capsaicin is marketed in the USA for topical treatment of arthritis (Medical Letter, 34:62, 1992). Some patients have found that continued use of the drug can relieve pain.

COMBINATION SECOND-LINE THERAPY — Combination therapy theoretically could be more effective than individual second-line agents due to additive effects and less toxic due to reduced individual drug dosages, but clinical trials have generally failed to show any added benefit (HJ Williams et al, Arthritis Rheum, 35:259, 1992;

RF Willkens et al, Arthritis Rheum, 35:849, 1992; KL Faarvang et al, Ann Rheum Dis, 52:711, 1993).

INVESTIGATIONAL DRUGS — Cyclosporine *(Sandimmune)* can be useful in some patients with refractory rheumatoid arthritis (RBM Landewe et al, J Rheumatol, 21:1631, 1994; GS Panayi and P Tugwell, Br J Rheumatol, 33:967, 1994). The antibiotic minocycline (*Minocin*, and others) was more effective than placebo and well-tolerated in a double-blind trial in more than 200 adults with rheumatoid arthritis (BC Tilley et al, Ann Intern Med, 122:81, 1995). Preliminary data suggest that monoclonal antibodies to tumor necrosis factor might be effective (MG Elliott et al, Lancet, 344:1105 and 1125, 1994). Dietary manipulation, particularly supplementation with omega-3 fatty acids, has been reported to be helpful (J Kjeldsen-Kragh et al, J Rheumatol, 19:1531, 1992), as have oral administration of gammalinolenic acid and collagen from articular cartilage (LJ Leventhal et al, Ann Intern Med, 119:867, 1993; DE Trentham et al, Science, 261:1727, 1993).

CONCLUSION — When rheumatoid arthritis does not respond to an NSAID, Medical Letter consultants often add hydroxychloroquine for patients with mild arthritis or methotrexate if the disease is more severe. In the dosage used to treat rheumatoid arthritis, methotrexate is often effective and well tolerated. Some consultants do not wait for a response but add the second drug as soon as the diagnosis is well established in an effort to avoid joint destruction and disability.

COST OF SOME NONSTEROIDAL ANTI-INFLAMMATORY DRUGS

Drug	Usual dosage range for arthritis	Cost*
Aspirin, extended-release –		
average generic price	1600 mg bid	$ 13.49
(range: $9.64 to $17.10)		
Extended Release Bayer 8 Hour† (Sterling)	1300 mg tid	17.25
ZORprin (Boots)	1600 mg to 3200 mg bid	36.36
Aspirin, enteric-coated† –		
average generic price	975 mg qid	10.19
(range: $3.06 to $21.42)		
Bayer Enteric Aspirin†		21.31
Non-acetylated salicylates		
Magnesium salicylate – *Magan* (Savage)	1090 mg tid-qid	91.71
Choline salicylate – *Arthropan*† (Purdue Frederick)	4.8 to 7.2 grams/day divided	60.31
Choline magnesium salicylate –		
average generic price	3 grams/day	49.36
(range: $40.32 to $64.78)	in 1, 2 or 3 doses	
Trilisate (Purdue Frederick)**		86.89
Sodium salicylate† –		
average generic price	3.6 to 5.4 grams/day	5.26
(range: $2.79 to $7.65)	divided doses	
Salicylsalicylic acid (salsalate) –		
average generic price	3 to 4 grams/day	25.28
(range: $16.20 to $50.92)	in 2 or 3 doses	
Disalcid (3M)		61.99
Mono-Gesic (Central)		34.56
Diclofenac – *Voltaren* (Ciba-Geigy)	150 to 200 mg/day in 2 or 3 doses	69.54
Diflunisal – average generic price		
(range: $46.66 to $59.19)	500 to 1000 mg/day in 2 doses	51.23
Dolobid (MSD)		55.30
Fenoprofen – average generic price		
(range: $24.63 to $31.94)	300 to 600 mg tid-qid	29.47
Nalfon (Dista)		34.88
Flurbiprofen – *Ansaid* (Upjohn)	200 to 300 mg/day in 2, 3 or 4 doses	71.72

Drug	Usual dosage range for arthritis	Cost*
Ibuprofen‡ – average generic price (range: $4.20 to $15.30)	1200 to 3200 mg/day in 3 or 4 doses	$ 9.71
Motrin (Upjohn)		17.85
Rufen (Boots)		17.91
Indomethacin – average generic price (range: $3.99 to $22.10)	25 to 50 mg tid-qid	11.55
Indocin (MSD)		48.54
extended-release – average generic price (range: $25.25 to $38.97)	75 mg once/day or bid	30.92
Indocin SR (MSD)		43.98
Ketoprofen – average generic price (range: $72.56 to $82.98)	50 to 75 mg tid-qid	78.86
Orudis (Wyeth-Ayerst)		89.11
Oruvail (Wyeth-Ayerst)	200 mg once/day	66.04
Meclofenamate sodium – average generic price (range: $27.00 to $61.20)	200 to 400 mg/day in 3 or 4 doses	43.40
Meclomen (Parke-Davis)		88.94
Nabumetone – *Relafen* (SK Beecham)	1000 once/day to 2000 mg/day	61.32
Naproxen – average generic price (range: $40.23 to $60)	250 to 500 mg bid-tid	42.96
Naprosyn (Syntex)**		46.46
Naproxen sodium‡ – average generic price (range: $36 to 49.06)	275 mg or 550 mg bid	40.57
Anaprox (Syntex)		46.31
Oxaprozin – *Daypro* (Searle)	1200 mg once/day to 1800 mg/day	72.70
Piroxicam – average generic price (range: $32.13 to $72.41)	20 mg once/day	61.57
Feldene (Pfizer)		77.17
Sulindac – average generic price (range: $36 to $52.56)	150 to 200 mg bid	46.12
Clinoril (MSD)		58.41
Tolmetin – average generic price (range: $41.48 to $45.90)	600 to 1800 mg/day in 3 or 4 doses	43.70
Tolectin (McNeil)		57.65

* Cost to the pharmacist for 30 days' treatment with the lowest usual dosage, based on wholesale price (AWP) listings in *Drug Topics Red Book* 1995 and May *Update*.

** Also available as liquid formulation.

† Available without a prescription.

‡ Also available without prescription in a lower tablet strength.

COST OF SECOND-LINE DRUGS FOR RHEUMATOID ARTHRITIS

Drug	Usual dosage range for arthritis	Cost*
Hydroxychloroquine sulfate– *Plaquenil* (Sanofi Winthrop)	200 to 400 mg/day	$ 34.78
Methotrexate, oral – average generic price (range: $43.11 to $64.65)	10 to 15 mg/week	48.86
Rheumatrex (Lederle)		52.81
Methotrexate, injectable	10 to 15 mg/week	
powder (Immunex)		11.12
liquid (Immunex)		19.00
liquid (Chiron)		27.52
Folex PFS (Pharmacia)		60.80
Gold sodium thiomalate – *Myochrysine* (MSD)	50 mg/week	42.88
Aurothioglucose – *Solganal* (Schering)	50 mg/week	45.64
Auranofin – *Ridaura* (SK Beecham)	3 mg bid or 6 mg once	65.80
Sulfasalazine – average generic price (range: $12.89 to $23.94)	2 to 4 grams/day	17.52
Azulfidine Entabs (Pharmacia)		29.47
Penicillamine – *Cuprimine* (MSD)	500 to 750 mg/day	53.86
Depen (Wallace)		81.44
Azathioprine – *Imuran* (Burroughs Wellcome)	1.5 to 2.5 mg/kg/day	70.73

* Cost to the pharmacist for 30 days' treatment with the lowest usual dosage, based on wholesale price (AWP) listings in *Drug Topics Red Book* 1995 and May *Update*. Cost of injectable methotrexate is based on single use of the smallest vial available.

DRUGS FOR ASTHMA

Asthma is now considered a chronic inflammatory disorder of the airways, with inflammation caused by allergens or other stimuli leading to bronchial hyper-responsiveness and obstruction of airflow. The recent therapeutic emphasis, therefore, has been on use of anti-inflammatory drugs (RA Goldstein et al, Ann Intern Med, 121:698, 1994). The treatment of asthma in the hospital or emergency room is not included here.

INHALED CORTICOSTEROIDS – Regular use of an inhaled corticosteroid can suppress inflammation, decrease bronchial hyper-responsiveness and decrease symptoms in patients with chronic asthma. Addition of an inhaled corticosteroid can improve asthma not controlled by bronchodilators alone (E Dompeling et al, Ann Intern Med, 118:770, 1993). Many clinicians now use inhaled corticosteroids in patients with mild or moderate asthma as well as those with severe disease. With time, the dosage can sometimes be decreased with no loss of control, but discontinuing an inhaled corticosteroid may lead to a relapse of the disease (T Haahtela et al, N Engl J Med, 331:700, 1994).

Toxicity – Recommended doses of inhaled corticosteroids have generally been free of serious toxicity. Suppression of the hypothalamic-pituitary-adrenal axis can be detected if sufficiently sensitive tests are used, but generally has no clinical importance (PJ Barnes and S Pedersen, Am Rev Respir Dis, 148:S1, 1993). Slowing of growth may occur in some children (DG Tinkelman et al, Pediatrics, 92:64, 1993), but one meta-analysis found no effect on final adult height (DB Allen et al, J Allergy Clin Immunol, 93:967, 1994). Decreased bone mineral density has been reported in premenopausal women (M Ip et al, Chest, 105:1722, 1994). Dysphonia and oral or esophageal candidiasis can occur due to local deposition of the drug; use of a spacer device and rinsing the mouth after inhalation can decrease these effects.

ORAL CORTICOSTEROIDS — Oral or parenteral corticosteroids are the most effective drugs available for acute exacerbations of asthma unresponsive to bronchodilators. Even when an acute exacerbation responds to bronchodilators, many clinicians treat recovering patients for up to 10 days with oral corticosteroids, which decrease symptoms and may prevent relapse (KR Chapman et al, N Engl J Med, 324:788, 1991). Prolonged daily use of oral corticosteroids can cause glucose intolerance, weight gain, increased blood pressure, bone demineralization, cataracts, immunosuppression and decreased growth in children. Alternate-day use can decrease the incidence of these adverse effects.

CROMOLYN SODIUM ***(Intal)*** **AND NEDOCROMIL** ***(Tilade)*** — Cromolyn sodium has anti-inflammatory properties and can decrease airway hyper-responsiveness in some patients with asthma. The drug has no bronchodilating activity and is useful only for prophylaxis, but it has virtually no systemic toxicity. A trial of up to six weeks may be necessary to determine whether it is effective. Pretreatment with cromolyn can prevent or diminish bronchospasm induced by exercise or cold dry air, but less effectively than inhalation of a $beta_2$ agonist. Nedocromil is a chemically unrelated drug with similar clinical effectiveness (Medical Letter, 35:62, 1993). Both cromolyn and nedocromil are less effective than inhaled corticosteroids in patients with moderate or severe chronic asthma.

$BETA_2$ AGONISTS — Inhaled short-acting $beta_2$-selective adrenergic agonists are the most effective drugs available for treatment of acute bronchospasm and for prevention of exercise-induced asthma (ER McFadden, Jr and IA Gilbert, N Engl J Med, 330:1362, 1994). Twice-daily inhalation of salmeterol, a long-acting $beta_2$ adrenergic agonist, has been effective for maintenance treatment and may be especially useful in patients with nocturnal symptoms. Adding regular use of salmeterol to use of an inhaled corticosteroid appears to be more effective in controlling moderate asthma than raising the dose of the corticosteroid (AP Greening, Lancet, 344:219, 1994). Patients taking salmeterol regularly should use a short-acting $beta_2$ agonist PRN to control acute symptoms (Medical Letter, 36:37, 1994). Oral $beta_2$ agonists are less effective and have a slower onset of action than the same drugs given by inhalation, but oral syrup formulations may be useful for some young children with mild symptoms who cannot use an inhaler.

Toxicity – Albuterol, bitolterol, pirbuterol, terbutaline and salmeterol are relatively $beta_2$-selective in their action and produce more bronchodilation with fewer cardiovascular effects than older adrenergic drugs such as epinephrine, isoproterenol or metaproterenol. Nevertheless, tachycardia, palpitations and tremor can occur, and high doses can cause hypokalemia. Overuse of inhaled $beta_2$ agonists has been associated with an increase in mortality, but whether overuse caused worsening of the disease or vice-versa is not clear (S Suissa et al, Am J Respir Crit Care Med, 149:604, 1994). Increased bronchial hyper-responsiveness has been associated with regular, rather than PRN, use of $beta_2$ agonists, particularly with fenoterol, which is not available in the USA (MR Sears and DR Taylor, Drug Safety, 11:259, 1994). Although some studies have shown a decrease in protection against airway hyper-responsiveness with regular use of the long-acting $beta_2$ agonist salmeterol (D Cheung et al, N Engl J Med, 327:1198, 1992), others have found that regular use for up to six months was not associated with deterioration in control of the disease (GE D'Alonzo et al, JAMA, 271:1412, 1994; AP Greening et al, Lancet, 344:219, 1994). Some patients using salmeterol regularly have died suddenly (FN Finkelstein, N Engl J Med, 331:1314, 1994); whether these deaths were caused by the drug or the disease is unclear.

THEOPHYLLINE — Oral theophylline is a less potent bronchodilator than inhaled $beta_2$ agonists and has a slower onset of action. Although theophylline has limited usefulness for treatment of acute symptoms, the drug can decrease the frequency and severity of symptoms in patients with chronic asthma, especially nocturnal asthma, and can decrease oral steroid requirements in corticosteroid-dependent patients. Since theophylline clearance varies, measurement of theophylline serum concentrations can help determine optimal dosage.

Toxicity – Patients with asthma may benefit from theophylline serum concentrations of less than 10 μg/ml, with few adverse effects. At concentrations of 10 to 20 μg/ml, nausea, nervousness, headache and insomnia may occur. At serum concentrations higher than 20 μg/ml, vomiting, hypokalemia, hyperglycemia, tachycardia, cardiac arrhythmias, tremor, neuromuscular irritability and seizures can occur. Many other drugs used concurrently can cause either an increase or decrease in serum theophylline concentrations (*The Medical Letter Handbook of Adverse Drug Interactions*, 1995, page 270).

IPRATROPIUM — Ipratropium bromide *(Atrovent)*, an atropine derivative sometimes used as an adjunct for inhalation treatment of chronic obstructive pulmonary disease (Medical Letter, 29:71, 1987), is a slow-acting, relatively weak bronchodilator but generally has had no serious adverse effects. Although not approved by the US Food and Drug Administration for treatment of asthma, ipratropium has been useful particularly in older, nonatopic patients with chronic obstruction to airflow.

CHOICE OF DRUGS — Both children and adults with infrequent symptoms of asthma may require only intermittent use, as needed, of a short-acting inhaled $beta_2$-selective adrenergic agonist. Patients with only exercise-induced asthma can use a $beta_2$ agonist before exercise. Medical Letter consultants do not agree on how frequent or severe asthma has to be before they would prescribe regular use of inhaled corticosteroids, but such use (together with a short-acting $beta_2$ agonist to control acute symptoms) can suppress airway inflammation and decrease bronchial hyper-responsiveness. Overuse of short-acting $beta_2$ agonists (more than a canister a month, according to some clinicians) indicates that an anti-inflammatory drug should be added to the treatment regimen or, if one is already being used, that the dose should be increased. Some pediatricians favor a trial of cromolyn or nedocromil before prescribing regular use of inhaled corticosteroids for children.

Maintenance treatment with a long-acting $beta_2$ agonist such as salmeterol can control the symptoms of asthma; many Medical Letter consultants recommend salmeterol only for patients also using an inhaled corticosteroid regularly. Oral theophylline can suppress the symptoms of asthma, particularly nocturnal symptoms, but requires careful monitoring to avoid toxicity. A short course of oral corticosteroids can control severe acute asthma symptoms unresponsive to other drugs.

SOME DRUGS FOR AMBULATORY ASTHMA

Drug	Formulation	Initial dosage Adult	Initial dosage Child (≤ 40 kg)
ANTI-INFLAMMATORY DRUGS			
Corticosteroids			
Beclomethasone dipropionate *(Beclovent, Vanceril)*	metered-dose inhaler[1] (42 μg/puff)	2-4 puffs bid-qid	2 puffs qid or 4 puffs bid
Budesonide *(Pulmicort)*[2]	metered-dose inhaler[1] (50, 200 μg/puff) or *Turbuhaler* (100, 200, 400 μg/puff)	400-2400 μg divided bid-qid	200-400 μg bid
Flunisolide *(Aerobid)*	metered-dose inhaler[1] (250 μg/puff)	2-4 puffs bid	2 puffs bid
Triamcinolone acetonide *(Azmacort)*	metered-dose inhaler[1] (100 μg/puff)	2 puffs tid-qid or 4 puffs bid	1-2 puffs tid-qid or 4 puffs bid
Prednisone or prednisolone	oral tablets (5, 10, 20 mg) oral liquid *(Liquid Pred, Pediapred, Prelone)*	Acute: up to 50 mg/day x 5-14 days Chronic: up to 40 mg every other day[3]	Acute: 10-40 mg bid x 5-14 days Chronic: 20-40 mg every other day[3]

(continued)

1. An aerosol-holding chamber (spacer device) is often used with a metered-dose inhaler. The device acts as a reservoir for the aerosolized drug and decreases the need to coordinate inspiration with actuation of the inhaler. *Azmacort* has a built-in spacer.
2. Available in Canada and Europe; among corticosteroids in this list, budesonide probably has the most favorable ratio of topical to systemic glucocorticoid activity.
3. Single dose on alternate days; when controlled for a month, taper by 5-10 mg every two weeks to lowest dose that keeps patient symptom-free.

Drug	Formulation	Initial dosage Adult	Child (≤ 40 kg)
Cromolyn *(Intal)*	*Spinhaler*, powder (20 mg/capsule)	1 capsule qid	1 capsule qid
	metered-dose inhaler[1,4] (800 μg/puff)	2-4 puffs qid	2-4 puffs qid
	nebulized solution[5] (10 mg/ml)	20 mg qid	20 mg qid
Nedocromil *(Tilade)*	metered-dose inhaler[1] (1.75 mg/puff)	2 puffs qid	2 puffs qid
BRONCHODILATORS			
Beta$_2$-selective adrenergic drugs			
Albuterol (*Proventil, Ventolin,* and others)	metered-dose inhaler[1] (90 μg/puff)	2 puffs q4-6h PRN[6]	2 puffs q4-6h PRN[6]
	Rotacaps, powder inhaler (200 μg/capsule)	1-2 caps q4-6h PRN[6]	1-2 caps q4-6h PRN[6]
	nebulized solution[5] (5 mg/ml)	2.5 mg tid-qid PRN	0.1-0.15 mg/kg q4-6h PRN
	syrup or tablets	2-4 mg tid or qid PRN	0.1 mg/kg (max. 2 mg) q6-8h PRN
	extended-release tablets (*Repetabs, Volmax*)	4-8 mg q12h	0.1-0.2 mg/kg q12h
Bitolterol mesylate *(Tornalate)*	metered-dose inhaler[1] (370 μg/puff)	2-3 puffs q4-6h PRN[6]	2 puffs q4-6h PRN[6]
	nebulized solution[5] (2 mg/ml)	1.5-3.5 mg bid-qid PRN	1.5 mg bid-qid PRN
Pirbuterol *(Maxair, Maxair Autohaler)*	metered-dose inhaler[1] (200 μg/puff)	2 puffs q4-6h PRN[6]	2 puffs q4-6h PRN[6]

(continued)

4. According to some Medical Letter consultants, the metered-dose inhaler may deliver less drug to the lungs than the nebulized solution or capsule formulation.
5. Nebulized solutions may be more convenient for very young, very old and other patients unable to use pressurized aerosols, and higher drug doses can be used. More time is required to administer the drug, however, and the device is not usually portable.
6. Each puff should be separated by 1-3 minutes in patients with acute distress to improve deposition of the aerosol.

Drug	Formulation	Initial dosage Adult	Child (≤ 40 kg)
Salmeterol *(Serevent)*	metered-dose inhaler[1] (21 μg/puff)	2 puffs bid[7]	1-2 puffs bid[7]
Terbutaline *(Brethaire)*	metered-dose inhaler[1] (200 μg/puff)	2 puffs q4-6h PRN[6]	2 puffs q4-6h PRN[6]
(Brethine, Bricanyl)	tablets	2.5-5 mg tid	1.25-2.5 mg tid
Theophylline	extended-release capsules or tablets[8] (*Theo-Dur*, and others)	300-600 mg/day[9]	Less than one year: mg/kg/day=(0.2) (age in weeks) + 5[9] 1-9 years: 12-20 mg/kg/day[9] 9-12 years: 12-18 mg/kg/day[9] 12-16 years: 12-16 mg/kg/day[9]

7. Long-acting. Should not be used PRN to control acute symptoms.
8. Extended-release formulations may not be interchangeable.
9. Begin with low dose and increase at 3-4 day intervals, depending on clinical response and serum concentrations to determine if larger doses can be given safely (L Hendeles et al, J Pediatr, 120:177, 1992). Children's initial dosage should not exceed 600 mg/day.

COST OF SOME AEROSOLS FOR ASTHMA

Drug	Canister size (grams)	Contents (puffs)	Cost*
Beta-adrenergics			
Albuterol – *Proventil* (Schering-Plough)	17	200	$ 23.05
Ventolin (Allen & Hanburys)	17	200	23.05
*Ventolin Rotacaps***			27.19
Bitolterol – *Tornalate* (Dura)	16.4	300	34.28
Pirbuterol – *Maxair* (3M)	25.6	300	23.04
Salmeterol – *Serevent* (Allen & Hanburys)	13	120	47.95
Terbutaline – *Brethaire* (Geigy)	10.5	300	20.75
Corticosteroids			
Beclomethasone dipropionate –			
Beclovent (Allen & Hanburys)	16.8	200	30.01
Vanceril (Schering-Plough)	16.8	200	30.01
Flunisolide – *Aerobid* (Forest)	7	100	49.02
Triamcinolone acetonide – *Azmacort* (Rhône-Poulenc Rorer)	20	240	41.63
Cromolyn sodium – *Intal* (Fisons)	8.1	112	37.98
Intal Nebulizer Solution†			48.25
Nedocromil – *Tilade* (Fisons)	16.2	112	25.28

* Cost to the pharmacist, based on wholesale price (AWP) listings in *Drug Topics Red Book* 1995 and May *Update.*

** Each kit contains 100 (200 µg) capsules and a *Rotahaler* device.

† Available in 60-ampule packages; each 2-ml ampule contains 20 mg.

DRUGS OF CHOICE FOR CANCER CHEMOTHERAPY

The tables that follow list drugs used for treatment of cancer in the USA and Canada and their major adverse effects. The choice of drugs in Table I is based on the opinions of Medical Letter consultants. Some drugs are listed for indications for which they have not been approved by the US Food and Drug Administration. Anticancer drugs and their adverse effects are listed in Table II. Table III lists some investigational drugs, which may be available from the National Cancer Institute or from the manufacturer.

TABLE I – DRUGS OF CHOICE

Cancer	Drugs of choice	Some alternatives
Adrenocortical**	Mitotane Cisplatin	Doxorubicin, streptozocin, etoposide
Bladder*	*Local:* Instillation of BCG *Systemic:* Methotrexate + vinblastine + doxorubicin + cisplatin (MVAC) Cisplatin + methotrexate + vinblastine (CMV)	Instillation of mitomycin, doxorubicin or thiotepa Paclitaxel, substitution of carboplatin for cisplatin in combinations
Brain		
anaplastic astrocytoma*	Procarbazine + lomustine + vincristine	Carmustine, cisplatin
anaplastic oligodendroglioma*	Procarbazine + lomustine + vincristine	Carmustine, cisplatin
glioblastoma**	Carmustine or lomustine	Procarbazine, cisplatin
medulloblastoma	Vincristine + carmustine ± mechlorethamine ± methotrexate Mechlorethamine + vincristine + procarbazine + prednisone (MOPP) Vincristine + cisplatin ± cyclophosphamide	Etoposide

(continued)

* Chemotherapy has only moderate activity.
** Chemotherapy has only minor activity.

Cancer	Drugs of choice	Some alternatives
Brain *(continued)*		
primary central nervous system lymphoma	Methotrexate (high dose intravenous and/or intrathecal) ± cytarabine (intravenous and/or intrathecal) Cyclophosphamide + doxorubicin + vincristine + prednisone (CHOP)	
Breast	*Adjuvant*[1]: Cyclophosphamide + methotrexate + fluorouracil (CMF); Cyclophosphamide + doxorubicin ± fluorouracil (AC or CAF); Tamoxifen	
	Metastatic: Cyclophosphamide + methotrexate + fluorouracil (CMF) **or** Cyclophosphamide + doxorubicin ± fluorouracil (AC or CAF) for receptor-negative and/or hormone-refractory; Tamoxifen for receptor-positive and/or hormone-sensitive[2]	Paclitaxel; thiotepa + doxorubicin + vinblastine; mitomycin + vinblastine; mitomycin + methotrexate + mitoxantrone; fluorouracil by continuous infusion; Bone marrow transplant[3]
Cervix**	Cisplatin Ifosfamide with mesna Bleomycin + ifosfamide with mesna + cisplatin	Chlorambucil, vincristine, fluorouracil, doxorubicin, methotrexate, altretamine
Choriocarcinoma	Methotrexate ± leucovorin Dactinomycin	Methotrexate + dactinomycin + cyclophosphamide (MAC) Etoposide + methotrexate + dactinomycin + cyclophosphamide + vincristine

* Chemotherapy has only moderate activity.

** Chemotherapy has only minor activity.

1. Tamoxifen with or without chemotherapy is generally recommended for postmenopausal estrogen-receptor-positive, node-positive patients and chemotherapy with or without tamoxifen for premenopausal node-positive patients. Adjuvant treatment with chemotherapy and/or tamoxifen is recommended for node-negative patients with larger tumors or other adverse prognostic indicators.
2. Megestrol and other hormonal agents may be effective in some patients when tamoxifen fails.
3. After high-dose chemotherapy (Medical Letter, 34:79, 1992).

Cancer	Drugs of choice	Some alternatives
Colorectal*	*Adjuvant colon*[4]: Fluorouracil + levamisole; Fluorouracil + leucovorin *Metastatic:* Fluorouracil + leucovorin	*Hepatic metastases:* Intrahepatic-arterial floxuridine Mitomycin
Embryonal rhabdomyosarcoma[5]	Vincristine + dactinomycin ± cyclophosphamide Vincristine + ifosfamide with mesna + etoposide	Same + doxorubicin
Endometrial**	Megestrol or another progestin Doxorubicin + cisplatin ± cyclophosphamide	Fluorouracil, tamoxifen, altretamine
Esophageal*	Cisplatin + fluorouracil	Doxorubicin, methotrexate, mitomycin
Ewing's sarcoma[5]	Cyclophosphamide (or ifosfamide with mesna) + doxorubicin + vincristine (CAV) ± dactinomycin	CAV + etoposide
Gastric**	Fluorouracil ± leucovorin	Cisplatin, doxorubicin, etoposide, methotrexate + leucovorin, mitomycin
Head and neck, squamous cell*[6]	Cisplatin + fluorouracil Methotrexate	Bleomycin, carboplatin, paclitaxel
Islet cell**	Streptozocin + doxorubicin	Streptozocin + fluorouracil; chlorozotocin†; octreotide
Kaposi's sarcoma* (AIDS-related)	Etoposide or interferon alfa or vinblastine Doxorubicin + bleomycin + vincristine or vinblastine (ABV)	Vincristine, doxorubicin, bleomycin

† Available in the USA only for investigational use.

4. For rectal cancer, postoperative adjuvant treatment with fluorouracil plus radiation, preceded and followed by treatment with fluorouracil alone.
5. Drugs have major activity only when combined with surgical resection, radiotherapy or both.
6. The vitamin A analog isotretinoin *(Accutane)* can control pre-neoplastic lesions (leukoplakia) and decreases the rate of second primary tumors (SE Benner et al, J Natl Cancer Inst, 86:140, 1994).

Cancer	Drugs of choice	Some alternatives
Leukemias		
Acute lymphocytic leukemia (ALL)[7]	*Induction:* Vincristine + prednisone + asparaginase ± daunorubicin *CNS prophylaxis:* Intrathecal methotrexate ± systemic high-dose methotrexate with leucovorin ± intrathecal cytarabine ± intrathecal hydrocortisone	*Induction:* same ± high-dose methotrexate ± cytarabine; pegaspargase instead of asparaginase Teniposide or etoposide High-dose cytarabine
	Maintenance: Methotrexate + mercaptopurine Bone marrow transplant[3, 8]	*Maintenance:* same + periodic vincristine + prednisone
Acute myeloid leukemia (AML)[9]	*Induction:* Cytarabine + either daunorubicin or idarubicin *Post Induction:* High-dose cytarabine ± other drugs such as etoposide Bone marrow transplant[3]	Cytarabine + mitoxantrone High-dose cytarabine
Chronic lymphocytic leukemia (CLL)	Chlorambucil ± prednisone Fludarabine	Cladribine, cyclophosphamide, pentostatin, vincristine, doxorubicin
Chronic myeloid leukemia (CML)[10]		
Chronic phase	Bone marrow transplant[3] Interferon alfa Hydroxyurea	Busulfan
Accelerated[11]	Bone marrow transplant[3]	Hydroxyurea, busulfan
Blast crisis[11]	*Lymphoid:* Vincristine + prednisone + L-asparaginase + intrathecal methotrexate (± maintenance with methotrexate + 6-mercaptopurine) *Myeloid:* High-dose cytarabine + daunorubicin	Tretinoin† Amsacrine,† azacitidine† Vincristine ± plicamycin
Hairy cell leukemia	Pentostatin or cladribine	Interferon alfa, chlorambucil, fludarabine

7. High-risk patients (e.g., high counts, cytogenetic abnormalities, adults) may require additional drugs for induction, maintenance and "intensification" (use of additional drugs after achievement of remission). Additional drugs include cyclophosphamide, mitoxantrone and thioguanine. The results of one large controlled trial in the United Kingdom suggest that intensification may improve survival in all children with ALL (JM Chessells et al, Lancet, 345:143, 1995).
8. Patients with a poor prognosis initially or those who relapse after remission

Cancer	Drugs of choice	Some alternatives
Liver**	Doxorubicin Fluorouracil	Intrahepatic-arterial floxuridine or cisplatin
Lung, small cell (oat cell)	Cisplatin + etoposide (PE) Cyclophosphamide + doxorubicin + vincristine (CAV) PE alternated with CAV Cyclophosphamide + etoposide + cisplatin (CEP) Doxorubicin + cyclophosphamide + etoposide (ACE)	Ifosfamide with mesna + carboplatin + etoposide (ICE) Daily oral etoposide Etoposide + ifosfamide with mesna + cisplatin (VIP) Paclitaxel
Lung (non-small cell)**	Cisplatin + etoposide Cisplatin + vinblastine ± mitomycin Cisplatin + vinorelbine	Cisplatin + fluorouracil + leucovorin Carboplatin + paclitaxel
Lymphomas		
Hodgkin's[12]	Doxorubicin + bleomycin + vinblastine + dacarbazine (ABVD) ABVD alternated with MOPP Mechlorethamine + vincristine + procarbazine (± prednisone) + doxorubicin + bleomycin + vinblastine (MOP[P]-ABV)	Mechlorethamine + vincristine + procarbazine + prednisone (MOPP) Chlorambucil + vinblastine + procarbazine + prednisone ± carmustine Etoposide + vinblastine + doxorubicin Bone marrow transplant[3]

9. Some patients with acute promyelocytic leukemia have had complete responses to tretinoin. Such treatment can cause a toxic syndrome characterized primarily by fever and respiratory distress (RP Warrell, Jr et al, N Engl J Med, 329:177, 1993).
10. Allogeneic HLA-identical sibling bone marrow transplantation can cure 40% to 70% of patients with CML in chronic phase, 15% to 25% of patients with accelerated phase CML, and < 15% patients in blast crisis. Disease-free survival after bone marrow transplantation is adversely influenced by age > 50 years, duration of disease > 3 years from diagnosis, and use of one-antigen-mismatched or matched-unrelated donor marrow. Interferon alfa may be curative in patients with chronic phase CML who achieve a complete cytogenetic response (about 10%); it is the treatment of choice for patients > 50 years old with newly diagnosed chronic phase CML and for all patients who are not candidates for an allogeneic bone marrow transplant. Chemotherapy alone is palliative.
11. If a second chronic phase is achieved with any of these combinations, allogeneic bone marrow transplant should be considered. Bone marrow transplant in second chronic phase may be curative for 30% to 35% of patients with CML.
12. Limited-stage Hodgkin's disease (stages 1 and 2) is curable by radiotherapy. Disseminated disease (stages 3b and 4) requires chemotherapy. Some intermediate stages and selected clinical situations may benefit from both.

Cancer	Drugs of choice	Some alternatives
Lymphomas *(continued)*		
Non-Hodgkin's		
Burkitt's lymphoma	Cyclophosphamide + vincristine + methotrexate Cyclophosphamide + high-dose cytarabine ± methotrexate with leucovorin Intrathecal methotrexate or cytarabine	Ifosfamide with mesna Cyclophosphamide + doxorubicin + vincristine + prednisone (CHOP)
Diffuse large-cell lymphoma	Cyclophosphamide + doxorubicin + vincristine + prednisone (CHOP)	Dexamethasone sometimes substituted for prednisone Other combination regimens, which may include methotrexate, etoposide, cytarabine, bleomycin, procarbazine, ifosfamide and mitoxantrone Bone marrow transplant[3]
Follicular lymphoma	Cyclophosphamide or chlorambucil	Same ± vincristine and prednisone, ± etoposide Interferon alfa, cladribine, fludarabine Bone marrow transplant[3] Cyclophosphamide + doxorubicin + vincristine + prednisone (CHOP)
Melanoma**	Interferon alfa Dacarbazine	Carmustine, lomustine, cisplatin Dacarbazine + cisplatin + carmustine + tamoxifen Aldesleukin
Mycosis fungoides*	PUVA (psoralen + ultraviolet A) Mechlorethamine (topical) Interferon alfa Electron beam radiotherapy Methotrexate	Isotretinoin, topical carmustine, pentostatin, fludarabine, cladribine, photopheresis (extracorporeal photochemotherapy), chemotherapy as in non-Hodgkin's lymphoma

* Chemotherapy has only moderate activity.

** Chemotherapy has only minor activity.

Cancer	Drugs of choice	Some alternatives
Myeloma*	Melphalan (or cyclophosphamide) + prednisone Melphalan + carmustine + cyclophosphamide + prednisone + vincristine Dexamethasone + doxorubicin + vincristine (VAD) Vincristine + carmustine + doxorubicin + prednisone (VBAP)	Interferon alfa Bone marrow transplant[3] High-dose dexamethasone
Neuroblastoma*	Doxorubicin + cyclophosphamide + cisplatin + teniposide or etoposide Doxorubicin + cyclophosphamide Cisplatin + cyclophosphamide	Carboplatin, etoposide Bone marrow transplant[3]
Osteogenic sarcoma[5]*	Doxorubicin + cisplatin ± etoposide ± ifosfamide	Ifosfamide with mesna, etoposide, carboplatin, high-dose methotrexate with leucovorin Cyclophosphamide + etoposide
Ovary	Cisplatin (or carboplatin) + paclitaxel Cisplatin (or carboplatin) + cyclophosphamide (CP) ± doxorubicin (CAP)	Ifosfamide with mesna, paclitaxel, tamoxifen, melphalan, altretamine
Pancreatic**	Fluorouracil ± leucovorin	Gemcitabine†
Prostate	Leuprolide (or goserelin) ± flutamide	Estramustine ± vinblastine, aminoglutethimide + hydrocortisone, estramustine + etoposide, diethylstilbestrol, nilutamide†
Renal**	Aldesleukin Interferon alfa	Vinblastine, floxuridine
Retinoblastoma[5]*	Doxorubicin + cyclophosphamide ± cisplatin ± etoposide ± vincristine	Carboplatin, etoposide, ifosfamide with mesna
Sarcomas, soft tissue, adult*	Doxorubicin ± dacarbazine ± cyclophosphamide ± ifosfamide with mesna	Mitomycin + doxorubicin + cisplatin Vincristine, etoposide

Cancer	Drugs of choice	Some alternatives
Testicular	Cisplatin + etoposide ± bleomycin (PEB)	Vinblastine (or etoposide) + ifosfamide with mesna + cisplatin (VIP) Bone marrow transplant[3]
Wilms' tumor[5]	Dactinomycin + vincristine ± doxorubicin ± cyclophosphamide	Ifosfamide with mesna, etoposide, carboplatin

TABLE II — SOME ANTICANCER DRUGS AND HORMONES

Drug	Acute toxicity†	Delayed toxicity†
Aldesleukin (interleukin-2; *Proleukin* – Cetus Oncology)	**Fever**; **fluid retention**; **hypotension**; **respiratory distress;** rash; anemia; thrombocytopenia; nausea and vomiting; diarrhea; capillary leak syndrome; nephrotoxicity; myocardial toxicity; hepatotoxicity; erythema nodosum; neutrophil chemotactic defects	Neuropsychiatric disorders; hypothyroidism; nephrotic syndrome; possibly acute leukoencephalopathy; brachial plexopathy; bowel perforation
Altretamine (hexamethylmelamine; *Hexalen* – US Bioscience)	Nausea and vomiting	**Bone marrow depression;** CNS depression; peripheral neuropathy; visual hallucinations; ataxia; tremors; alopecia; rash
Aminoglutethimide (*Cytadren* – Ciba)	Drowsiness; nausea; dizziness; rash	Hypothyroidism (rare); bone marrow depression; fever; hypotension; masculinization

† Dose-limiting effects are in bold type. Cutaneous reactions (sometimes severe), hyperpigmentation, and ocular toxicity have been reported with virtually all nonhormonal anticancer drugs. For adverse interactions with other drugs, see *The Medical Letter Handbook of Adverse Drug Interactions*, 1995.

Drug	Acute toxicity[†]	Delayed toxicity[†]
Asparaginase (*Elspar* – Merck; *Kidrolase* in Canada)	Nausea and vomiting; fever; chills; headache; hypersensitivity, anaphylaxis; abdominal pain; hyperglycemia leading to coma	CNS depression or hyperexcitability; acute hemorrhagic pancreatitis; coagulation defects; thrombosis; renal damage; hepatic damage
BCG (*TheraCys* – Connaught; *Tice BCG* – Organon)	Bladder irritation; nausea and vomiting; fever; sepsis	Granulomatous pyelonephritis; hepatitis; urethral obstruction; epididymitis; renal abscess
Bleomycin (*Blenoxane* – Bristol-Myers Oncology)	Nausea and vomiting; fever; anaphylaxis and other allergic reactions; phlebitis at injection site	**Pneumonitis and pulmonary fibrosis**; rash and hyperpigmentation; stomatitis; alopecia; Raynaud's phenomenon; cavitating granulomas; hemorrhagic cystitis
Busulfan (*Myleran* – Burroughs Wellcome)	Nausea and vomiting; rare diarrhea	**Bone marrow depression; pulmonary infiltrates and fibrosis**; alopecia; gynecomastia; ovarian failure; hyperpigmentation; azoospermia; leukemia; chromosome aberrations; cataracts; hepatitis; seizures and veno-occlusive disease with high doses
Carboplatin (*Paraplatin* – Bristol-Myers Oncology)	Nausea and vomiting	**Bone marrow depression**; peripheral neuropathy (uncommon); hearing loss; transient cortical blindness; hemolytic anemia
Carmustine (BCNU; *BiCNU* – Bristol-Myers Oncology)	Nausea and vomiting; local phlebitis	**Delayed leukopenia and thrombocytopenia** (may be prolonged); pulmonary fibrosis (may be irreversible); delayed renal damage; reversible liver damage; leukemia; myocardial ischemia
Chlorambucil (*Leukeran* – Burroughs Wellcome)	Nausea and vomiting; seizures	**Bone marrow depression**; pulmonary infiltrates and fibrosis; leukemia; hepatic toxicity; sterility

Drug	Acute toxicity†	Delayed toxicity†
Cisplatin (Cis-DDP; *Platinol* – Bristol-Myers Oncology)	Nausea and vomiting; diarrhea; anaphylactic reactions	**Renal damage**; ototoxicity; bone marrow depression; hemolysis; hypomagnesemia; peripheral neuropathy; hypocalcemia; hypokalemia; Raynaud's disease; sterility; hypophosphatemia; hyperuricemia
Cladribine (2-chlorodeoxy-adenosine; CdA; *Leustatin* – Ortho-Biotech)	Fever	**Bone marrow depression**; peripheral neuropathy with high doses
Cyclophosphamide (*Cytoxan* – Mead Johnson Oncology, *Procytox* in Canada)	Nausea and vomiting; Type I (anaphylactoid) hypersensitivity; facial burning with IV administration; visual blurring	**Bone marrow depression**; alopecia; hemorrhagic cystitis; sterility (may be temporary); pulmonary infiltrates and fibrosis; hyponatremia; leukemia; bladder cancer; inappropriate ADH secretion; cardiac toxicity
Cytarabine HCl (*Cytosar-U* – Upjohn, and others)	Nausea and vomiting; diarrhea; anaphylaxis; sudden respiratory distress with high doses	**Bone marrow depression**; conjunctivitis; megaloblastosis; oral ulceration; hepatic damage; fever; pulmonary edema and central and peripheral neurotoxicity with high doses; rhabdomyolysis; pancreatitis when used with asparaginase; rash
Dacarbazine (*DTIC-Dome* – Miles, and others)	Nausea and vomiting; diarrhea; anaphylaxis; pain on administration	**Bone marrow depression**; alopecia; flu-like syndrome; renal impairment; hepatic necrosis; facial flushing; paresthesia; photosensitivity; urticarial rash

† Dose-limiting effects are in bold type. Cutaneous reactions (sometimes severe), hyperpigmentation, and ocular toxicity have been reported with virtually all nonhormonal anticancer drugs. For adverse interactions with other drugs, see *The Medical Letter Handbook of Adverse Drug Interactions*, 1995.

Drug	Acute toxicity[†]	Delayed toxicity[†]
Dactinomycin (*Cosmegen* – Merck)	Nausea and vomiting; hepatic toxicity with ascites; diarrhea; severe local tissue damage and necrosis on extravasation; anaphylactoid reaction	**Stomatitis; oral ulceration; bone marrow depression**; alopecia; folliculitis; dermatitis in previously irradiated areas
Daunorubicin HCl (*Cerubidine* – Wyeth-Ayerst, Rhône-Poulenc Rorer in Canada)	Nausea and vomiting; diarrhea; red urine (not hematuria); severe local tissue damage and necrosis on extravasation; transient EKG changes; facial flushing; anaphylactoid reaction	**Bone marrow depression; cardiotoxicity** (may be delayed for years); alopecia; stomatitis; anorexia; diarrhea; fever and chills; dermatitis in previously irradiated areas; skin and nail pigmentation
Diethylstilbestrol (Lilly; *Stilphostrol* – Miles)	Nausea and vomiting; abdominal cramps; headache	Gynecomastia in males; breast tenderness; loss of libido; thrombophlebitis and thromboembolism; hepatic injury; sodium retention with edema; hypertension; change in menstrual flow
Doxorubicin HCl (*Adriamycin* – Pharmacia, and others)	Nausea and vomiting; red urine (not hematuria); severe local tissue damage and necrosis on extravasation; diarrhea; fever; transient EKG changes; ventricular arrhythmia; anaphylactoid reaction	**Bone marrow depression; cardiotoxicity** (may be delayed for years); alopecia; stomatitis; anorexia; conjunctivitis; acral pigmentation; dermatitis in previously irradiated areas; acral erythrodysesthesia; hyperuricemia
Estramustine phosphate sodium (*Emcyt* – Pharmacia)	Nausea and vomiting; diarrhea	Mild gynecomastia; increased frequency of vascular accidents; myelosuppression (uncommon); edema; dyspnea; pulmonary infiltrates and fibrosis; decreased glucose tolerance; thrombosis; hypertension

Drug	Acute toxicity†	Delayed toxicity†
Etoposide (VP16-213; *VePesid* – Bristol-Myers Oncology)	Nausea and vomiting; diarrhea; fever; hypotension; anaphylactoid reactions; phlebitis at infusion site	**Bone marrow depression**; rashes; alopecia; peripheral neuropathy; mucositis and hepatic damage with high doses; leukemia
Etretinate (*Tegison* – Roche)		Dryness of mucous membranes; chapped lips; hair loss; bone and joint pain; eye irritation; peeling skin; pseudotumor cerebri; premature epiphyseal closure; hepatic injury; major teratogenic effects
Finasteride (*Proscar* – Merck)		Impotence; decreased libido; teratogenic
Floxuridine (*FUDR* – Roche, and others)	Nausea and vomiting; diarrhea	**Oral and gastrointestinal ulceration**; **bone marrow depression**; alopecia; dermatitis; hepatic dysfunction with hepatic infusion
Fludarabine (*Fludara* – Berlex)	Nausea and vomiting	**Bone marrow depression;** CNS effects; visual disturbances; renal damage with higher doses; pulmonary infiltrates; tumor lysis syndrome
Fluorouracil (5-FU; *Adrucil* – Pharmacia, and others)	Nausea and vomiting; diarrhea; hypersensitivity reaction (rare)	**Oral and GI ulcers**; **bone marrow depression**; diarrhea (especially with fluorouracil and leucovorin); neurological defects, usually cerebellar; cardiac arrhythmias; angina pectoris; alopecia; hyperpigmentation; palmar-plantar erythrodysesthesia; conjunctivitis; heart failure; seizures

† Dose-limiting effects are in bold type. Cutaneous reactions (sometimes severe), hyperpigmentation, and ocular toxicity have been reported with virtually all nonhormonal anticancer drugs. For adverse interactions with other drugs, see *The Medical Letter Handbook of Adverse Drug Interactions*, 1995.

Drug	Acute toxicity†	Delayed toxicity†
Flutamide (antiandrogen; *Eulexin* – Schering, *Euflex* in Canada)	Nausea; diarrhea	Gynecomastia; hepatotoxicity
Gallium nitrate (*Ganite* – Solo Pak)	Hypocalcemia	**Hypophosphatemia;** nephrotoxicity; anemia
Goserelin (*Zoladex* – Zeneca)	Transient increase in bone pain and ureteral obstruction in patients with metastatic prostate cancer; hot flashes	Impotence; testicular atrophy; gynecomastia
Hydroxyurea (*Hydrea* – Bristol-Myers Oncology)	Nausea and vomiting; allergic reactions to tartrazine dye	**Bone marrow depression**; stomatitis; dysuria; alopecia; rare neurological disturbances; pulmonary infiltrates
Idarubicin (*Idamycin* – Pharmacia)	Nausea and vomiting; tissue damage on extravasation	**Bone marrow depression;** alopecia; stomatitis; myocardial toxicity; diarrhea
Ifosfamide (*Ifex* – Mead Johnson Oncology)	Nausea and vomiting; confusion; nephrotoxicity; metabolic acidosis and renal Fanconi's syndrome; **cardiac toxicity** with high doses	**Bone marrow depression**; **hemorrhagic cystitis** (prevented by concurrent mesna); alopecia; inappropriate ADH secretion; renal failure; neurotoxicity (somnolence, hallucinations, blurring of vision, coma)
Interferon alfa-2a, alfa-2b, alfa-n3 (*Roferon-A* – Roche, *Intron A* – Schering, *Alferon N* – Purdue Frederick)	Fever; chills; myalgias; fatigue; headache; arthralgias; hypotension	Bone marrow depression; anorexia; neutropenia; anemia; confusion; depression; renal toxicity; possible hepatic injury; facial and peripheral edema; cardiac arrhythmias
Isotretinoin (*Accutane* – Roche)	Fatigue; headache; nausea and vomiting; pruritus	**Teratogenicity; cheilitis;** xerostomia; rash; conjunctivitis and eye irritation; bone and joint pain; anorexia; hypertriglyceridemia; pseudotumor cerebri

Drug	Acute toxicity†	Delayed toxicity†
Leuprolide acetate (LHRH-analog; *Lupron, Lupron Depot* – TAP)	Transient increase in bone pain and ureteral obstruction in patients with metastatic prostate cancer; hot flashes	Impotence; testicular atrophy; CNS effects; gynecomastia; peripheral edema
Levamisole (*Ergamisol* – Janssen)	Nausea and vomiting; diarrhea; flu-like symptoms; metallic taste	Agranulocytosis; arthralgias; rash; encephalopathy; hyperlipidemia; pancreatitis; fatigue; peripheral neuropathy
Lomustine (CCNU; *CeeNU* – Bristol-Myers Oncology)	Nausea and vomiting	**Delayed (4 to 6 weeks) leukopenia and thrombocytopenia** (may be prolonged); transient elevation of transaminase activity; neurological reactions; pulmonary fibrosis; renal damage; leukemia
Mechlorethamine HCl (nitrogen mustard; *Mustargen* – Merck)	**Nausea and vomiting**; local reaction and phlebitis	**Bone marrow depression**; alopecia; diarrhea; oral ulcers; leukemia; amenorrhea; sterility; hyperuricemia
Medroxyprogesterone acetate (*Provera, Depo-Provera* – Upjohn, and others)	Nausea; urticaria; headache; fatigue	Menstrual changes; gynecomastia; hot flashes; weight gain; hirsutism; insomnia; fatigue; depression; edema; thrombophlebitis and thromboembolism; sterile abscess
Megestrol acetate (*Megace* – Mead Johnson Oncology, and others)	Nausea and vomiting; headache	Menstrual changes; hot flashes; thrombophlebitis and thromboembolism; fluid retention; edema; weight gain
Melphalan (*Alkeran* – Burroughs Wellcome)	Mild nausea; hypersensitivity reactions	**Bone marrow depression** (especially platelets); pulmonary infiltrates and fibrosis; amenorrhea; sterility; leukemia

† Dose-limiting effects are in bold type. Cutaneous reactions (sometimes severe), hyperpigmentation, and ocular toxicity have been reported with virtually all nonhormonal anticancer drugs. For adverse interactions with other drugs, see *The Medical Letter Handbook of Adverse Drug Interactions*, 1995.

Drug	Acute toxicity†	Delayed toxicity†
Mercaptopurine (*Purinethol* – Burroughs Wellcome)	Nausea and vomiting; diarrhea	**Bone marrow depression**; cholestasis and rarely hepatic necrosis; oral and intestinal ulcers; pancreatitis
Mesna (*Mesnex* – Bristol-Myers Oncology; *Uromitexan* in Canada)	Nausea and vomiting; diarrhea; allergic reactions	
Methotrexate (MTX; *Folex* – Pharmacia, and others)	Nausea and vomiting; diarrhea; fever; anaphylaxis; hepatic necrosis	**Oral and gastrointestinal ulceration**, perforation may occur; **bone marrow depression**; hepatic toxicity including cirrhosis; renal toxicity; **pulmonary infiltrates and fibrosis**; osteoporosis; conjunctivitis; alopecia; depigmentation; menstrual dysfunction; encephalopathy; infertility; lymphoma
Mitomycin (*Mutamycin* – Bristol-Myers Oncology)	Nausea and vomiting; tissue necrosis; fever	**Bone marrow depression** (cumulative); stomatitis; alopecia; acute pulmonary toxicity; pulmonary fibrosis; hepatotoxicity; renal toxicity; amenorrhea; hemolytic-uremic syndrome; bladder calcification (with intravesical administration)
Mitotane (o,p'-DDD; *Lysodren* – Bristol-Myers Oncology)	Nausea and vomiting; diarrhea	**CNS depression**; rash; visual disturbances; adrenal insufficiency; hematuria; hemorrhagic cystitis; albuminuria; hypertension; orthostatic hypotension; cataracts; prolonged bleeding time
Mitoxantrone HCl (*Novantrone* – Immunex)	Blue-green pigment in urine; blue-green sclera; nausea and vomiting; stomatitis; fever; phlebitis	**Bone marrow depression**; cardiotoxicity; alopecia; white hair; skin lesions; hepatic damage; renal failure; extravasation necrosis

Drug	Acute toxicity†	Delayed toxicity†
Octreotide (*Sandostatin* – Sandoz)	Nausea and vomiting; diarrhea	Steatorrhea; gallstones
Paclitaxel (*Taxol* – Mead Johnson Oncology)	Anaphylaxis, dyspnea, hypotension, angioedema, urticaria (probably due to vehicle)	**Bone marrow depression**; peripheral neuropathy; alopecia; arthralgias; myalgias; cardiac toxicity; mild GI disturbances; mucositis
Pegaspargase (PEG-L-asparaginase; *Oncaspar* – Rhône-Poulenc Rorer)	Similar to asparaginase	Similar to asparaginase
Pentostatin (2'-deoxycoformycin; *Nipent* – Parke-Davis)	Nausea and vomiting; rash	Nephrotoxicity; CNS depression; **bone marrow depression**; respiratory failure; hepatic toxicity; arthralgia; myalgia; photophobia; conjunctivitis
Plicamycin (*Mithracin* – Miles)	Nausea and vomiting	**Hemorrhagic diathesis**; thrombocytopenia; coagulation abnormalities; hepatic damage; hypocalcemia; renal damage
Procarbazine HCl (*Matulane* – Roche, *Natulan* in Canada)	Nausea and vomiting; CNS depression; disulfiram-like effect with alcohol; adverse interactions typical of a monoamine oxidase (MAO) inhibitor	**Bone marrow depression**; stomatitis; peripheral neuropathy; pneumonitis; leukemia
Streptozocin (*Zanosar* – Upjohn, and others)	Nausea and vomiting; local pain	**Renal damage**; hypoglycemia; hyperglycemia; liver damage; diarrhea; bone marrow depression (uncommon); fever; eosinophilia; nephrogenic diabetes insipidus

† Dose-limiting effects are in bold type. Cutaneous reactions (sometimes severe), hyperpigmentation, and ocular toxicity have been reported with virtually all nonhormonal anticancer drugs. For adverse interactions with other drugs, see *The Medical Letter Handbook of Adverse Drug Interactions*, 1995.

Drug	Acute toxicity†	Delayed toxicity†
Tamoxifen citrate (*Nolvadex* – Zeneca, and others; *Tamofen* in Canada)	Hot flashes; nausea and vomiting; transient increased bone or tumor pain; hypercalcemia	Vaginal bleeding and discharge; rash; thrombocytopenia; peripheral edema; depression; dizziness; headache; decreased visual acuity; corneal changes; retinopathy; purpuric vasculitis; thromboembolism; endometrial cancer
Teniposide (VM-26; *Vumon* – Bristol-Myers Oncology)	Nausea and vomiting; diarrhea; phlebitis; anaphylactoid symptoms	**Bone marrow depression**; alopecia; peripheral neuropathy; leukemia
Thioguanine (Burroughs Wellcome, *Lanvis* in Canada)	Occasional nausea and vomiting; diarrhea	**Bone marrow depression**; hepatic damage; stomatitis
Thiotepa (Immunex)	Nausea and vomiting; rare hypersensitivity reaction	**Bone marrow depression**; menstrual dysfunction; interference with spermatogenesis; leukemia; mucositis with high doses
Trimetrexate (*Neutrexin* – US Bioscience)	Fever; chills; nausea and vomiting; diarrhea	**Bone marrow depression; mucositis**; peripheral neuropathy; rash; pruritus; hyperpigmentation; nephrotoxicity; hepatic injury
Vinblastine sulfate (*Velban* – Lilly, and others; *Velbe* in Canada)	Nausea and vomiting; local reaction and tissue damage with extravasation	**Bone marrow depression**; alopecia; stomatitis; loss of deep tendon reflexes; jaw pain; muscle pain; paralytic ileus
Vincristine sulfate (*Oncovin* – Lilly, and others)	Tissue damage with extravasation	**Peripheral neuropathy**; alopecia; mild bone marrow depression; constipation; paralytic ileus; jaw pain; inappropriate ADH secretion; optic atrophy
Vinorelbine tartrate (*Navelbine* – Burroughs Wellcome)	Nausea and vomiting; diarrhea; constipation; dyspnea; injection site reactions (erythema, discoloration, phlebitis, pain)	**Bone marrow depression**; alopecia; anorexia; stomatitis; asthenia; peripheral neuropathy

TABLE III — SOME INVESTIGATIONAL DRUGS

Drug	Acute toxicity*	Delayed toxicity*
**Amsacrine (m-AMSA; amsidine; *AMSA P-D* – Parke-Davis, *Amsidyl* – Warner-Lambert)	Nausea and vomiting; diarrhea; pain or phlebitis on infusion; anaphylaxis	**Bone marrow depression**; hepatic injury; convulsions; stomatitis; ventricular fibrillation; alopecia; congestive heart failure; renal dysfunction
Azacitidine (ladakamycin; *Mylosar* – Upjohn)	Nausea and vomiting; diarrhea; fever; rash; drowsiness	**Bone marrow depression**; hepatic damage; muscle pain and weakness; possibly cardiotoxicity
Chlorozotocin (DCNU – Dome)	Similar to streptozocin, but less nausea and vomiting	Similar to streptozocin, but **leukopenia** and **thrombocytopenia** are common
Gemcitabine (*Gemzar* – Lilly)	Fatigue	Bone marrow depression
**Nilutamide (*Anandron* – Roussel Uclaf)	Nausea and vomiting, alcohol intolerance	Delayed adaptation to darkness; interstitial pneumonitis; hepatic toxicity
Tretinoin (*Vesanoid* – Roche)	**Headache; xerosis**; pruritus; "retinoic acid syndrome" (fever, dyspnea, pulmonary infiltrates, pleural effusions, peripheral edema, hypotension); arthralgias; myalgias	**Cheilitis; teratogenicity;** rashes; leucocytosis; hypertriglyceridemia; pseudotumor cerebri; thrombophlebitis

* Dose-limiting effects are in bold type. Cutaneous reactions (sometimes severe), hyperpigmentation, and ocular toxicity have been reported with virtually all nonhormonal anticancer drugs. For adverse interactions with other drugs, see *The Medical Letter Handbook of Adverse Drug Interactions*, 1995.

** Commercially available in Canada.

PARTIAL LIST OF BRAND NAMES

Accutane – isotretinoin
**Adriamycin* – doxorubicin
**Adrucil* – fluorouracil
Alferon N – interferon alfa-n3
Alkeran – melphalan
†*AMSA P-D* – amsacrine
Anandron – nilutamide
†*Amsidyl* – amsacrine
BiCNU – carmustine
Blenoxane – bleomycin
CeeNU – lomustine
Cerubidine – daunorubicin
Cosmegen – dactinomycin
Cytadren – aminoglutethimide
**Cytosar-U* – cytarabine
**Cytoxan* – cyclophosphamide
Depo-Provera – medroxyprogesterone acetate
**DTIC-Dome* – dacarbazine
**Efudex* – fluorouracil
Elspar – asparaginase
Emcyt – estramustine phosphate sodium
Ergamisol – levamisole
Euflex – flutamide
Eulexin – flutamide
Fludara – fludarabine
**Fluoroplex* – fluorouracil
**Folex* – methotrexate
**FUDR* – floxuridine
Ganite – gallium nitrate
†*Gemzar* – gemcitabine
Hexalen – altretamine
Hydrea – hydroxyurea
Idamycin – idarubicin
Ifex – ifosfamide
Intron-A – interferon alfa-2b
Kidrolase – asparaginase
Lanvis – thioguanine
Leukeran – chlorambucil
Leustatin – cladribine
Lupron – leuprolide acetate
Lysodren – mitotane
Matulane – procarbazine
**Megace* – megestrol acetate
Mesnex – mesna
Mithracin – plicamycin
Mustargen – mechlorethamine
Mutamycin – mitomycin
Myleran – busulfan
†*Mylosar* – azacitidine
Navelbine – vinorelbine tartrate
Natulan – procarbazine
**Neosar* – cyclophosphamide
Neutrexin – trimetrexate
Nipent – pentostatin
Nolvadex – tamoxifen citrate
Novantrone – mitoxantrone
Oncaspar – pegaspargase
**Oncovin* – vincristine sulfate
†*Pharmorubicin* – epirubicin
Platinol – cisplatin
**Procytox* – cyclophosphamide
Proleukin – (interleukin-2) aldesleukin
Proscar – finasteride
Provera – medroxyprogesterone acetate
Purinethol – mercaptopurine
Roferon-A – interferon alfa-2a
**Rubex* – doxorubicin
Sandostatin – octreotide
Stilphostrol – diethylstilbestrol
Tamofen – tamoxifen
Tamone – tamoxifen
**Tarabine* – cytarabine
Taxol – paclitaxel
Tegison – etretinate
TheraCys – BCG live
Tice BCG – BCG vaccine
Uromitexan – mesna
**Velbe* – vinblastine
**Velban* – vinblastine
VePesid – etoposide
†*Vesanoid* – tretinoin
**Vincasar* – vincristine
Vumon – teniposide
**Zanosar* – streptozocin
Zoladex – goserelin

---

* Also available generically
† Investigational in USA

DRUGS FOR CARDIAC ARRHYTHMIAS

Several approaches have been proposed to classify drugs used for treatment of cardiac arrhythmias based on the premise that drugs with similar electrophysiologic properties are also similar in their therapeutic effects and cardiac toxicity. Agents that appear to be similar in the laboratory, however, may have many different effects in patients. In practice, the choice of drugs is based mainly on clinical experience, especially with cardiac and noncardiac toxicity. Some of the drugs listed in the table on page 57 are recommended for indications for which they have not been approved by the US Food and Drug Administration.

The dosages, adverse effects and therapeutic serum concentrations of each drug are given in the table that begins on page 60. Antiarrhythmic drugs may themselves cause arrhythmias, which can be fatal. Several studies have indicated that some antiarrhythmic agents, given to asymptomatic or mildly symptomatic patients, increase rather than decrease mortality (DM Roden, N Engl J Med, 331:785, 1994).

BETA-ADRENERGIC BLOCKERS — Beta-blockers can control the ventricular rate in atrial fibrillation or flutter and terminate regular supraventricular tachycardias. They are also safer, although somewhat less effective, than other drugs for suppression of symptomatic VPCs. Beta-blockers are usually well tolerated, but can cause bradyarrhythmias, bronchospasm, impotence, mood alterations, fatigue or worsening of congestive heart failure. Sudden withdrawal of a beta-blocker in a patient with angina pectoris can precipitate increasing angina, a cardiac arrhythmia or a myocardial infarction. Four drugs in this class have been approved by the US Food and Drug Administration for treatment of various arrhythmias: **propranolol** (*Inderal*, and others), **acebutolol** (*Sectral* – Medical Letter, 27:58, 1985), **sotalol** (*Betapace* – Medical Letter, 35:27, 1993), and **esmolol** (*Brevibloc* – Medical Letter, 29:57, 1987).

Sotalol is not only a beta-blocker, but also blocks potassium channels, prolonging repolarization (see page 55). Esmolol is an intravenous cardioselective agent with an elimination half-life of about nine minutes; it is effective in controlling the ventricular response in atrial flutter or fibrillation, particularly after cardiac surgery, and both therapeutic and adverse effects (hypotension, bradycardia) usually disappear within 30 minutes after stopping an infusion. **Atenolol** (*Tenormin*, and others) and **metoprolol** *(Lopressor)* have been associated with decreased mortality in the first week after myocardial infarction; chronic administration of propranolol, metoprolol, or **timolol** (*Blocadren*, and others) has decreased long-term mortality after myocardial infarction.

CALCIUM-CHANNEL BLOCKERS — **Verapamil** (*Calan*, and others) and **diltiazem** *(Cardizem)* prolong AV refractoriness and are effective in terminating many re-entrant supraventricular tachycardias and slowing the ventricular rate in atrial fibrillation or flutter. Their intravenous use can be complicated by hypotension or bradycardia, especially with concurrent use of other cardiodepressant drugs, in patients with underlying heart disease or in those with ventricular tachycardia, in whom these drugs are ineffective and can be dangerous. Verapamil is also approved for chronic oral supraventricular antiarrhythmic therapy. Both verapamil and diltiazem are generally contraindicated in patients with atrial fibrillation associated with the Wolff-Parkinson-White syndrome. Either verapamil or diltiazem can elevate serum digoxin concentrations, and both interact with many other drugs (*The Medical Letter Handbook of Adverse Drug Interactions*, 1995, pages 126 and 292). **Bepridil** (*Vascor* – Medical Letter, 33:53, 1991) is a calcium-channel blocker that also prolongs the QT interval; it has antiarrhythmic properties, but can also cause polymorphic ventricular tachycardia with excessive QT prolongation (torsades de pointes). Usual doses of calcium-channel blockers of the dihydropyridine subclass (all those available in the USA except for verapamil, diltiazem and bepridil) have no antiarrhythmic activity.

QUINIDINE, PROCAINAMIDE, DISOPYRAMIDE — **Quinidine** is usually given orally as the sulfate or gluconate; sustained-release preparations may be erratically absorbed. The dosage required to achieve therapeutic serum concentrations varies markedly from one patient to another. The gluconate can also be given intravenously (IV), but adverse effects, particularly hypotension, are more frequent with parenteral use. When quinidine is given to a patient with atrial fibrillation or especially with atrial flutter, the ventricular rate may increase as the atrial rate slows; an AV-nodal blocking agent such as digoxin, verapamil or a beta-blocker is usually given first. Quinidine can, however, increase digoxin concentrations to potentially toxic levels, and also interacts with many other drugs (*The Medical Letter Handbook of Adverse Drug Interactions*, 1995, page 245). Torsades de pointes is the likely cause of "quinidine syncope," a syndrome that can occur even with low serum concentrations or even after single doses of quinidine and is potentiated by hypokalemia, hypomagnesemia and bradycardia. The results of some studies have suggested that use of quinidine in some patients with atrial fibrillation may increase mortality (GC Flaker et al, J Am Coll Cardiol, 20:527, 1992; SE Coplen et al, Circulation, 82:1106, 1990).

Procainamide (*Pronestyl*, and others) can be given IV more safely than quinidine, although hypotension can occur with rapid loading doses. With long-term use, adverse extracardiac effects, such as fever or rash, occur commonly. Many patients develop antinuclear antibodies (ANA) after three to six months of therapy, and 15% to 20% develop a lupus-like syndrome, which disappears slowly when the drug is discontinued. Agranulocytosis unrelated to the lupus reaction occurs in 0.5% of patients. Plasma concentrations of procainamide and NAPA, its active metabolite, may be increased in renal failure or by concurrent use of amiodarone *(Cordarone)*, cimetidine *(Tagamet)*, ranitidine *(Zantac)*, or trimethoprim (*Trimpex*, and others) (*The Medical Letter Handbook of Adverse Drug Interactions*, 1995, page 241).

Disopyramide (*Norpace*, and others) can aggravate heart failure, and anticholinergic effects are often prominent; urinary retention frequently requires discontinuation of the drug. Nevertheless, in some patients it may be tolerated better than quinidine.

FLECAINIDE, PROPAFENONE, MORICIZINE — **Flecainide** *(Tambocor)*, and **propafenone** *(Rythmol)* markedly decrease the rate of cardiac conduction, but only modestly increase the ventricular refractory period (Medical Letter, 28:19, 1986; 32:37, 1990). **Moricizine** (*Ethmozine* – Medical Letter, 32:99, 1990) also slows conduction but has little effect on repolarization. Although all three are effective in suppressing ventricular arrhythmias, they also can aggravate existing arrhythmias or precipitate new ones, especially in patients with underlying heart disease and sustained ventricular tachycardia. Use of flecainide, encainide (no longer marketed) or moricizine in a clinical trial in post-myocardial infarction patients with asymptomatic ventricular arrhythmias was associated with an increase in mortality compared to placebo (AE Epstein et al, JAMA, 270:2451, 1993). Whether propafenone, which unlike flecainide or moricizine also has beta-blocking activity, would have the same effect is unknown.

ADENOSINE — An intravenous drug, adenosine *(Adenocard)* is highly effective in terminating many supraventricular arrhythmias (LI Ganz and PL Friedman, N Engl J Med, 332:162, 1995). Although it can cause hypotension or transient atrial fibrillation, adenosine is probably safer than verapamil or diltiazem because it disappears from the circulation within seconds. Because of its safety, many cardiologists now prefer adenosine over a calcium-channel blocker for termination of sustained supraventricular tachycardia. As with calcium-channel blockers or digoxin, patients with Wolff-Parkinson-White syndrome and atrial fibrillation may develop ventricular proarrhythmias when given standard doses of adenosine (DV Exner et al, Ann Intern Med, 122:351, 1995).

LIDOCAINE AND SIMILAR AGENTS — **Lidocaine** (*Xylocaine*, and others), which is only given IV, is mainly metabolized by the liver. Patients with heart failure or with decreased hepatic function or hepatic blood flow and those more than 70 years old should, therefore, receive lower loading and maintenance doses. Clearance of the drug often changes during therapy; monitoring plasma concentrations can decrease toxicity. At serum concentrations above 5 μg/ml, central-nervous-system (CNS) depression, stimulation or seizures may occur; severe reactions are often preceded by tinnitus, slurred speech, somnolence, confusion or paresthesias. Propranolol or cimetidine (*Tagamet*, and others) can decrease the clearance of lidocaine, and concurrent use of tocainide or mexiletine can cause additive CNS toxicity, including seizures. The practice of giving lidocaine prophylactically to patients with suspected acute myocardial infarction has largely been abandoned because clinical trials failed to show a reduction in mortality.

Mexiletine *(Mexitil)* and **tocainide** *(Tonocard)* are orally effective congeners of lidocaine used to treat symptomatic ventricular arrhythmias. Nausea and tremor are common with both, but are less severe when the drugs are taken with food. Tocainide is rarely indicated because of adverse hematological effects, including a 0.2% incidence of agranulocytosis; it should be reserved for symptomatic patients who have not responded to other drugs, and blood counts should be monitored. Concurrent use of mexiletine or tocainide with quinidine may control arrhythmias at lower doses and with fewer adverse effects than with either drug used alone. The anticonvulsant agent **phenytoin** (*Dilantin*, and others) has similar electrophysiologic properties and has been used with inconsistent results to treat ventricular arrhythmias, except for digitalis-induced tachyarrhythmias, where the rate of success has been higher.

AMIODARONE AND SOTALOL — Amiodarone *(Cordarone)* has generally been reserved in the USA for oral treatment of life-threatening ventricular arrhythmias refractory to other antiarrhythmic agents; patients taking the drug should be monitored closely (Medical Letter, 28:49, 1986). Recent data suggest it may be superior to "conventional" drugs such as quinidine or procainamide for serious ventricular arrhythmias (The Cascade Investigators, Am J Cardiol, 72:280, 1993). Amiodarone can suppress VPCs and nonsustained ventricular tachycardia and prevent recurrences of sustained ventricular tachycardia or fibrillation. Doses of the drug lower than those used routinely have been used successfully to treat patients with recurrent supraventricular arrhythmias (DL Disch et al, Ann Intern Med, 120:449, 1994). Some studies have suggested that amiodarone may decrease the incidence of sudden death after an acute myocardial infarction (L Ceremuzynski et al, J Am Coll Cardiol, 20:1056, 1992), while others have failed to show such an effect; large randomized trials evaluating amiodarone are nearing completion. Low doses of the drug have been reported to improve contractility in patients with heart failure (HC Doval et al, Lancet, 344:493, 1994). Severe adverse effects, including pulmonary toxicity, can occur with usual doses of amiodarone and may be lethal or irreversible or persist for months after treatment is stopped. Low doses appear to cause fewer adverse effects (PJ Podrid, Ann Intern Med, 122:689, 1995). Amiodarone can increase the serum concentrations, pharmacological effects and toxicity of digoxin, diltiazem, quinidine, procainamide, flecainide, beta-blockers, oral anticoagulants and phenytoin (*The Medical Letter Handbook of Adverse Drug Interactions*, 1995, page 21). An intravenous formulation is likely to be available soon in the USA for patients with recurrent sustained ventricular tachycardia or fibrillation. Phlebitis, hypotension and exacerbation of heart failure are the major adverse effects of intravenous amiodarone.

Sotalol *(Betapace)* is a non-selective beta-blocker that also prolongs the QT interval. It is widely used outside the USA for treatment of supraventricular and ventricular arrhythmias (SH Hohnloser and RL Woosley, N Engl J Med, 331:31, 1994). The results of one study suggest that sotalol, like amiodarone, may be more effective than "conventional" agents in the treatment of serious ventricular arrhythmias, its only approved indication in the USA (JW Mason, N Engl J Med, 329:452, 1993). Major adverse effects are those related to beta-blockade and the torsades de pointes ventricular arrhythmia which, in contrast to quinidine, is a dose-related effect of sotalol.

OTHER AGENTS — Bretylium (*Bretylol*, and others; *Bretylate* in Canada) given intravenously can stabilize cardiac rhythm in about 50% of patients with resistant ventricular fibrillation or recurrent ventricular tachycardia refractory to other treatment. **Digoxin** (*Lanoxin*, and others) can control ventricular response in atrial fibrillation or flutter and may terminate some regular (reentrant) supraventricular arrhythmias. Digoxin, like verapamil and diltiazem, is generally contraindicated in patients in atrial fibrillation with the Wolff-Parkinson-White syndrome. Intravenous **magnesium** appears effective in preventing recurrent torsades de pointes (D Tzivoni, Circulation, 77:392, 1988) and in some arrhythmias related to digitalis toxicity. Results of a recent large trial indicate that intravenous magnesium administered to patients with a suspected myocardial infarction does not decrease mortality (ISIS-4, Lancet, 345:669, 1995).

NONPHARMACOLOGIC APPROACHES — Radiofrequency (RF) catheter ablation is a technique in which small areas of tissue responsible for the genesis or maintenance of some arrhythmias can be identified and destroyed. RF ablation is more than 90% effective in preventing recurrences of most regular supraventricular tachycardias such as AV nodal re-entry or arrhythmias related to the Wolff-Parkinson-White syndrome (RK Thakur, Can Med Assoc J, 151:771, 1994). Serious complications, which are rare, include inadvertent complete AV nodal ablation (usually requiring permanent pacing) and cardiac perforation (which may require emergency surgery). RF ablation has also "cured" some cases of atrial flutter or sustained ventricular tachycardia and controlled ventricular rate in atrial fibrillation, but is still being evaluated for these indications. **Implantable cardioverter/defibrillators (ICDs)** can be used in some patients who have survived an episode of sustained ventricular tachycardia or fibrillation (Medical Letter, 36:86, 1994). Trials are now underway comparing treatment with ICDs to antiarrhythmic agents such as amiodarone, sotalol or metoprolol (HL Greene, Am Heart J, 127:1171, 1993).

DRUGS OF CHOICE FOR COMMON ARRHYTHMIAS

Arrhythmia	Drug of choice	Alternatives	Remarks
Atrial fibrillation or flutter[1]	Verapamil, diltiazem or a beta-blocker to slow ventricular response	Digoxin to slow ventricular response Quinidine, procainamide, disopyramide, flecainide, propafenone or sotalol for long-term suppression	Digoxin, verapamil, diltiazem and possibly beta-blockers may be dangerous for patients with Wolff-Parkinson-White syndrome. Amiodarone in low doses has also been effective for suppression. Clonidine can also slow the ventricular response[2]
Other supraventricular tachycardias[3]	Adenosine, verapamil[4] or diltiazem[4] for termination	Esmolol, another beta-blocker or digoxin for termination	Cardioversion or atrial pacing may be effective for some patients. Radiofrequency catheter ablation can "cure" many patients. Quinidine, procainamide, disopyramide, diltiazem, beta-blockers, verapamil, flecainide, propafenone or digoxin may be effective for long-term suppression.

(continued)

1. Electrical cardioversion is the treatment of choice for recent onset with compromised circulation due to an excessively rapid ventricular rate. For patients with atrial flutter, atrial pacing can also be effective. Patients with Wolff-Parkinson-White syndrome and atrial fibrillation should be treated with IV procainamide if hemodynamically stable and, if not, with electrical cardioversion.
2. A Roth et al, Ann Intern Med, 116:338, 1992.
3. Vagotonic maneuvers (such as carotid sinus massage, gagging, the Valsalva maneuver, or increasing venous return by straight leg raising) may be tried first.
4. Verapamil and diltiazem are contraindicated for patients receiving intravenous beta-blockers or those with congestive heart failure and should be used with caution in patients taking oral quinidine.

Arrhythmia	Drug of choice	Alternatives	Remarks
Ventricular premature complexes (VPCs) or non-sustained ventricular tachycardia	No drug therapy indicated for asymptomatic patients	For symptomatic patients, a beta-blocker	There is no evidence that prolonged suppression with drugs prevents sudden cardiac death. For post-MI patients, treatment with a beta-blocker has decreased mortality, and treatment with flecainide or moricizine has increased it.
Sustained ventricular tachycardia[5,6]	Lidocaine for acute treatment	IV procainamide, bretylium	Cardioversion is the safest and most effective therapy. Sotalol, other beta-blockers, procainamide, quinidine, amiodarone, disopyramide, flecainide, propafenone or mexiletine may be effective for long-term suppression.[7]
Ventricular fibrillation[8]	Lidocaine	IV procainamide, amiodarone, bretylium	See footnote 7
Cardiac glycoside-induced ventricular tachyarrhythmias[6,9]	Digoxin-immune Fab (digoxin antibody fragments – *Digibind*)	Lidocaine, phenytoin	Self-limited if short-acting digitalis stopped. Phenytoin can also be effective. Avoid cardioversion and bretylium, except for ventricular fibrillation or sustained ventricular tachycardia. A beta-blocker or procainamide can make heart block worse.

5. Electrical cardioversion is preferred by most cardiologists for sustained ventricular tachycardia causing hemodynamic compromise, but some first try a chest thump, IV lidocaine or both.
6. Some ventricular tachycardias can be caused or exacerbated by bradycardia or heart block. In the presence of high-grade heart block, antiarrhythmic drugs can cause cardiac standstill. When high-grade heart block is present, therefore, a temporary pacemaker should be inserted before using antiarrhythmic drugs; pacing may abolish the arrhythmia. When a drug must be used in the presence of heart block, lidocaine is least likely to increase the block.
7. Specialized techniques such as programmed stimulation of the heart may be required to select long-term therapy, and some patients may be candidates for implanted cardioverter/defibrillators (Medical Letter, 36:86, 1994).

Arrhythmia	Drug of choice	Alternatives	Remarks
Torsades de pointes	Magnesium sulfate	Cardiac pacing, isoproterenol	Causative agents (e.g., quinidine) should be discontinued. Magnesium may be effective even in absence of hypomagnesemia. Potassium should be used to elevate serum K to between 4 and 5.5 mEq/L[9]

8. Defibrillation is the treatment of choice; drugs are for prevention of recurrence.
9. KCl can be given carefully, 10-20 mEq/hr IV, to patients with low or normal serum potassium concentrations. Extreme care must be taken to keep serum potassium below 5.5 mEq/L. In the presence of heart block not associated with paroxysmal atrial tachycardia, potassium should be withheld if the serum concentration is greater than 4.0 to 4.5 mEq/L, since high serum potassium may increase atrioventricular block.

DOSAGE AND ADVERSE EFFECTS OF ANTIARRHYTHMIC DRUGS

Drug	Usual dosage* and interval	Effect on ECG
BETA-ADRENERGIC BLOCKERS		
Propranolol (*Inderal*, and others)	PO: 10-80 mg q6h (long-acting formulation available) IV: 1-5 mg total (1 mg/min)	Prolongs PR (±) No Change QRS Bradycardia
Acebutolol *(Sectral)*	PO: 200 mg bid, increase gradually to 600-1200 mg/day	Bradycardia
Esmolol *(Brevibloc)*	IV Loading: 500 μg/kg over one minute, followed by 50 μg/kg/min; titrate to desired effect Usual maintenance: 100 μg/kg/min; maximum 300 μg/kg/min	Sinus bradycardia
CALCIUM-CHANNEL BLOCKERS		
Verapamil HCl (*Calan*, and others)	IV Initial dose: 5-10 mg over 2-3 min; repeat in 15-30 min, if necessary IV Infusion: Initial dose is followed by 0.375 mg/min for 30 min IV Maintenance: 0.125 mg/min PO: 40-120 mg tid or qid (long-acting formulation available)	Prolongs PR Sinus bradycardia
Diltiazem *(Cardizem)*	IV Initial dose: 0.15-0.35 mg/kg (10-25 mg) over 2 min, may be repeated in 15-30 min IV infusion: 5-15 mg/hr	Prolongs PR Sinus bradycardia
QUINIDINE, PROCAINAMIDE, DISOPYRAMIDE		
Quinidine (many manufacturers)	PO: 200-400 mg q4-6h (sulfate) 324-648 mg q8-12h (gluconate)	Prolongs QRS, QT and (±) PR
Procainamide (*Pronestyl*, and others)	PO: 50-100 mg/kg/day in divided doses, q3-4h or q6h (sustained-release) IV Loading: 20 mg/min (up to 17 mg/kg) IV Maintenance: 2-4 mg/min	Prolongs QRS, QT and (±) PR

* Patients with decreased hepatic or renal function may require lower dosage.

† Range of usually effective and tolerated concentrations

Adverse effects	Serum concentrations[†]
Heart block, hypotension, heart failure, bronchospasm, depression	Not useful
Hypotension, bradycardia, bronchospasm, ANA, arthritis, myalgia, arthralgia, lupus-like syndrome, pulmonary complications	Not established
Hypotension, heart block, heart failure, bronchospasm, pain at infusion site	0.15 to 2 μg/ml
Heart block, heart failure, hypotension, asystole, dizziness, headache, fatigue, edema, nausea, constipation	Not clinically useful
Heart block, hypotension, asystole, heart failure, liver damage	Not clinically useful
Diarrhea and other GI symptoms, cinchonism, hepatic granulomas and necrosis, thrombocytopenia, rashes, hypotension, heart block, tachyarrhythmias, torsades de pointes, fever, lupus-like syndrome	1.5 to 5 μg/ml
Lupus-like syndrome, confusion, disorientation, GI symptoms, rash, hypotension, arrhythmias, torsades de pointes, blood dyscrasias, fever, rare muscular weakness IV: hypotension, heart block	4 to 10 μg/ml (NAPA active metabolite: 7 to 15 μg/ml)

(continued)

Drug	Usual dosage* and interval	Effect on ECG
Disopyramide (*Norpace*, and others)	PO: 100-200 mg q6-8h or 150-300 mg q12h (long-acting formulation)	Prolongs QRS, QT and (±) PR
FLECAINIDE, PROPAFENONE, MORICIZINE		
Flecainide *(Tambocor)*	PO Initial dose: 50-100 mg q12h, increase q4 days if required, by 50 mg q12h PO Maintenance: ≤400 mg/day (≤300 mg for SVT)	Prolongs PR and QRS
Propafenone *(Rythmol)*	PO Initial dose: 150 mg q8h, increase q3-4 days if required PO Maintenance: 150 to 300 mg q8h	Prolongs PR and QRS
Moricizine *(Ethmozine)*	PO Initial dose: 200 mg q8h, increase by 150 mg/day q3-4 days if required PO Maintenance: 200-300 mg q8h	Prolongs PR and QRS
ADENOSINE		
Adenosine *(Adenocard)*	IV: 6 mg; may use 6-12 mg for repeat rapid bolus injection	Prolongs PR Heart block (transient)
LIDOCAINE AND SIMILAR AGENTS		
Lidocaine (*Xylocaine*, and others)	IV Loading: 1 mg/kg given over 2 min, then 0.5 mg/kg over 2 min every 8-10 min x 3 *or*: 20 mg/min infused over 10 min IV Maintenance: 1-4 mg/min	No significant change
Mexiletine *(Mexitil)*	PO Initial dose: 150-200 mg q8h taken with food PO Maintenance: 150-300 mg q6-12h, maximum 1200 mg/day	No significant change

* Patients with decreased hepatic or renal function may require lower dosage.
† Range of usually effective and tolerated concentrations
** Not reliable due to saturable protein binding

Adverse effects	Serum concentrations[†]
Anticholinergic effects (urinary retention, aggravation of glaucoma, constipation), hypotension, heart failure, tachyarrhythmias, torsades de pointes, heart block, nausea, vomiting, diarrhea, hypoglycemia, nervousness	2 to 5 μg/ml**
Bradycardia, heart block, new ventricular fibrillation, sustained ventricular tachycardia, heart failure, dizziness, blurred vision, nervousness, headache, GI upset, neutropenia	0.2 to 1 μg/ml
Bradycardia, heart block, new ventricular fibrillation, sustained ventricular tachycardia, heart failure, dizziness, lightheadedness, metallic taste, GI upset, bronchospasm, hepatic toxicity	Not established due to active metabolites
Bradycardia, heart failure, new ventricular fibrillation, sustained ventricular tachycardia, nausea, dizziness, headache	Not established due to active metabolites
Facial flushing, transient dyspnea, chest discomfort (non-coronary), hypotension; may cause bronchoconstriction in patients with asthma	Not established
Drowsiness or agitation, slurred speech, tinnitus, disorientation, coma, seizures, paresthesias, cardiac depression, especially with excessive accumulation in heart failure or liver failure or infusions for more than 24 hours, bradycardia/asystole	1.5 to 5 μg/ml
GI upset, fatigue, nervousness, dizziness, tremor, sleep upset, seizures, visual disturbances, psychosis, fever, blood dyscrasias, hepatitis	0.5 to 2 μg/ml

(continued)

Drug	Usual dosage* and interval	Effect on ECG
Tocainide *(Tonocard)*	PO Initial dose: 200-400 mg q8h with food PO Maintenance: 200-600 mg q8h, maximum 2400 mg/day	No significant change
AMIODARONE AND SOTALOL		
Amiodarone *(Cordarone)*	PO Loading: 800-1600 mg/day for 1-3 weeks then 600-800 mg/day for 4 weeks PO Maintenance: 100-400 mg/day IV Rapid loading: 150 mg over 10 minutes, which can be repeated once if needed IV Slow loading: 360 mg over 6 hours IV Maintenance: 540 mg over 18 hours	Prolongs PR, QRS and QT Sinus bradycardia
Sotalol *(Betapace)*	80-160 mg twice daily (Higher doses can be used, but may be associated with increased adverse effects including torsades de pointes)	Prolongs QT Sinus bradycardia
OTHER AGENTS		
Bretylium (*Bretylol*, and others; *Bretylate* in Canada)	IV Loading: 5 mg/kg with additional doses of 10 mg/kg to maximum of 30 mg/kg (effect may be delayed) IV Maintenance: 5-10 mg/kg q6h or continuous infusion 1-2 mg/min	No change Sinus bradycardia
Digoxin (*Lanoxin*, and others)	IV or PO Loading: 1-1.5 mg over 24 hours in 3-4 divided doses Maintenance: 0.125-0.5 mg/day	Prolongs PR Depresses ST segment Flattens T wave

* Patients with decreased hepatic or renal function may require lower dosage.

† Range of usually effective and tolerated concentrations

Adverse effects	Serum concentrations†
GI upset, paresthesias, dizziness, tremor, confusion, nightmares, psychotic reactions, coma, seizures, rash, fever, arthralgia, agranulocytosis, aplastic anemia, thrombocytopenia, hepatic granulomas, interstitial pneumonitis	3 to 10 μg/ml
Acute pulmonary toxicity, pulmonary fibrosis, bradycardia, heart block, new ventricular fibrillation, sustained ventricular tachycardia, torsades de pointes (unusual), hyper- or hypothyroidism, GI upset, alcoholic-like hepatitis, peripheral neuropathy, ataxia, tremor, dizziness, photosensitivity, blue-gray skin, corneal microdeposits	1 to 2 μg/ml (usefulness for monitoring toxicity unclear)
Heart block, hypotension, bronchospasm, bradycardia, torsades de pointes	0.5-1.0 μg/ml for beta-blockade, higher for QT effect (generally not clinically useful)
Orthostatic hypotension, nausea and vomiting, increased sensitivity to catecholamines, initial increase in arrhythmias	Not established
Bradycardia, AV block, arrhythmias, anorexia, nausea, vomiting, diarrhea, abdominal pain, headache, confusion, abnormal vision	1-2 ng/ml

CHOICE OF CHOLESTEROL-LOWERING DRUGS

Lowering elevated plasma cholesterol concentrations can slow progression, cause regression and prevent formation of new atherosclerotic lesions; it can also improve coronary vasodilatation (CB Treasure et al, N Engl J Med, 332:481, 1995; TJ Anderson et al, N Engl J Med, 332:488, 1995). Most authorities advise patients with high cholesterol concentrations to eat less fat, especially saturated fat, eat less cholesterol and, when appropriate, to increase physical activity and lose weight (Expert Panel, JAMA, 269:3015, 1993). If these measures do not lower plasma lipids sufficiently, drugs are frequently added to the regimen. When drugs are discontinued, plasma cholesterol concentrations generally return to pretreatment levels.

LIPOPROTEINS, TRIGLYCERIDES AND APOLIPOPROTEINS — Most of the cholesterol in plasma is carried in low-density lipoproteins (LDL); high plasma concentrations of LDL are associated with an increased risk of coronary heart disease. High plasma concentrations of high-density lipoproteins (HDL) are associated with a reduced risk of coronary heart disease. Triglycerides are carried in the plasma mainly in very-low-density lipoproteins (VLDL); they may also play a role in the pathogenesis of coronary atherosclerosis (R Havel, Curr Opin Lipidol, 5:102, 1994). Apolipoproteins are protein constituents of lipoproteins. High concentrations of apolipoprotein B (the main structural protein of LDL) and of lipoprotein(a) have been associated with an increased risk of coronary artery disease (AM Scanu et al, Ann Intern Med, 115:209, 1991; J Genest, Jr et al, J Am Coll Cardiol, 19:792, 1992).

HMG-CoA REDUCTASE INHIBITORS — Pravastatin *(Pravachol)*, simvastatin *(Zocor)* and fluvastatin (*Lescol* – Medical Letter, 36:45, 1994) are relatively new inhibitors of cholesterol synthesis similar to lovastatin *(Mevacor)*.

Effect on Plasma Cholesterol – All of these drugs inhibit HMG-CoA (3-hydroxy-3-methyl-glutaryl-coenzyme A) reductase, the enzyme that catalyzes the rate-limiting step in cholesterol synthesis; they are more effective than other types of drugs in lowering plasma concentrations of LDL and total cholesterol. They also reduce levels of triglycerides and VLDL cholesterol and may increase HDL cholesterol. Comparative studies have shown that 10 mg per day of simvastatin and 20 mg of pravastatin or lovastatin produce equivalent reductions of LDL-cholesterol in primary hypercholesterolemia (DR Illingworth et al, Lancet, 343:1554, 1994). While maximal fluvastatin dosage (40 mg per day) decreased LDL-cholesterol by 24% (RI Levy et al, Circulation, 87:III-45, 1993), maximum doses of lovastatin (80 mg), pravastatin (40 mg) and simvastatin (40 mg) generally decrease LDL by about 30% to 40% (ML Larsen and DR Illingworth, Med Clin North Am, 8S:225, 1994). Preliminary reports of direct comparisons of lovastatin and simvastatin with fluvastatin appear to confirm these differences (ML Berger et al; DR Illingworth et al; L Ose; 64th Congress of the European Atherosclerosis Society, June 10-13, 1995). When these drugs are taken once a day, it should be in the evening because the highest rate of cholesterol synthesis occurs between midnight and 3 a.m.; their effectiveness decreases when taken in the morning.

Effect on Mortality – A placebo-controlled, randomized trial compared simvastatin, 20 or 40 mg daily, with placebo in 4,444 diet-treated men and women with moderate hypercholesterolemia (213 to 310 mg/dl) and with a history of angina pectoris or acute myocardial infarction. After 4.3 to 6.3 years, 256 (12%) of the patients in the placebo group and 182 (8%) of the patients who took simvastatin had died, a statistically significant difference. The difference in mortality was due entirely to a reduction in coronary deaths; non-cardiovascular mortality was unaffected (Scandinavian Simvastatin Survival Study Group, Lancet, 344:1383, 1994).

Effect on Atherosclerosis – Placebo-controlled studies of lovastatin, simvastatin and pravastatin in patients with coronary atherosclerosis on angiography have shown that active treatment for two to four years slowed the progression and, in some studies, caused regression of coronary lesions (DH Blankenhorn et al, Ann

Intern Med, 119:969, 1993; MAAS Investigators, Lancet, 344:633, 1994; JW Jakema et al, Circulation, 91:2528, 1995). Controlled trials of lovastatin and pravastatin in men and women have also shown slower progression or regression of atherosclerosis in the carotid artery (CD Furberg et al, Circulation, 90:1679, 1994; JR Crouse III et al, Am J Cardiol, 75:445, 1995).

Adverse Effects – HMG-CoA reductase inhibitors are generally better tolerated than other cholesterol-lowering drugs. Mild, transient gastrointestinal disturbances, muscle pain, rash and headache have been the most common adverse effects, and some patients have reported sleep disturbances, occasionally associated with anxiety and irritability. An increase in plasma aminotransferase activities to more than three times normal occurs in 1% to 2% of patients taking higher doses of these drugs and may require discontinuation, but symptomatic hepatitis has been rare. A lupus-like syndrome has been reported with both lovastatin and simvastatin (S Ahmad, Arch Intern Med, 151:1667, 1991; B Bannwarth et al, Arch Intern Med, 152:1093, 1992), and peripheral neuropathy has been reported with both lovastatin and pravastatin. Both an increased hypoprothombinemic effect and bleeding have been reported when lovastatin was given together with oral anticoagulants (*The Medical Letter Handbook of Adverse Drug Interactions*, 1995, p 177).

Myopathy – Severe myalgia or muscle weakness with more than ten-fold increases in serum creatine phosphokinase concentrations has been reported rarely with all four drugs. Hepatic disease, severe infections, renal failure, hypothyroidism, advanced age and concurrent treatment with gemfibrozil *(Lopid)*, erythromycin or, rarely, niacin have increased the incidence of myopathy. Cyclosporine *(Sandimmune)* can also increase the incidence of myopathy, but apparently not with pravastatin. Rarely, myoglobinuria has led to acute renal failure.

Long Term – Cholesterol itself is a component of all human cell membranes; the long-term consequences of interfering indefinitely with its synthesis and the synthesis of related compounds are unknown. In controlled trials with up to six years' follow-up, patients treated with these drugs have had no detectable increase in the incidence of cancer, and the drugs were generally well tolerated. A recent study found discontinuation rates of less than 20% for lovastatin, while the rates for bile acid sequestrants, niacin and gemfibrozil were more than 35% (SE Andrade et al, N Engl J Med, 332:1125, 1995).

CHOLESTYRAMINE AND COLESTIPOL — The bile acid-binding resins cholestyramine *(Questran; Questran Light)* and colestipol *(Colestid)* lower concentrations of LDL cholesterol. A 7- to 10-year double-blind randomized trial compared the effects of cholestyramine with placebo in 3,806 men without known coronary artery disease but with a baseline plasma cholesterol of at least 265 mg/dl; all patients followed a moderate cholesterol-lowering diet. After seven years, the incidence of nonfatal myocardial infarction or death from coronary heart disease was 8.6% in the placebo-treated patients and 7% in the cholestyramine group; overall mortality was not affected (The Lipid Research Clinics Primary Prevention Trial, JAMA, 251:351, 1984). A six-year post-trial follow-up showed similar mortality rates for cancer, other medical causes and trauma in the two treatment groups, but total mortality was about 8% lower (143 vs 156) in cholestyramine-treated patients (The Lipid Research Clinics Investigators, Arch Intern Med, 152:1399, 1992). In an angiographic study, 90 men with coronary heart disease were assigned at random to usual care, diet or diet plus cholestyramine. After 39 months, both diet and diet plus cholestyramine decreased the percentage of patients with progressive coronary narrowing and increased the percentage with coronary widening; the increase in the coronary lumen was greater with cholestyramine (GF Watts et al, Lancet, 339:563, 1992).

Adverse Effects – The adverse effects of colestipol and cholestyramine are similar; constipation occurs frequently and may be accompanied by heartburn, nausea, belching and bloating, but these symptoms tend to disappear over time. Giving the drugs in moderate doses (8 to 10 grams daily or less) just before meals improves tolerance, and increased dietary fiber or a fiber supplement, such as psyllium (*Metamucil*, and others), may relieve constipation and bloating. Both cholestyramine and colestipol may interfere with absorption of fat-soluble vitamins and many other drugs; this can be avoided by giving other drugs either two hours before or four to six hours after the bile sequestering agent (*The Medical Letter Handbook of Adverse Drug Interactions*, 1995, pages 99 and 105). Plasma concentrations of triglycerides may rise, especially in patients with hypertriglyceridemia.

NIACIN (NICOTINIC ACID) — Although the mechanism is not known, niacin decreases triglycerides, total serum cholesterol and LDL cholesterol, and increases HDL cholesterol (JM King et al, Am J Med, 97:323, 1994). It also lowers lipoprotein(a), except in patients with severe hypertriglyceridemia. In one placebo-controlled trial, men with one or more previous myocardial infarctions who took niacin had a lower incidence of nonfatal myocardial infarction and, nine years later, a lower mortality rate (PL Canner et al, J Am Coll Cardiol, 8:1245, 1986).

Adverse Effects – Niacin can cause flushing, pruritus and gastrointestinal distress, but these problems can be relieved by taking aspirin before the first dose of the day (some patients require it more often) and can be minimized by taking a low initial dosage, increasing it gradually, taking the drug with meals and avoiding concurrent intake of hot beverages or alcohol. Niacin can also cause blurred vision, fatigue, glucose intolerance, hyperuricemia, exacerbation of peptic ulcer and, rarely, dry eyes or hyperpigmentation. Hepatic toxicity, sometimes severe, has been reported mainly with sustained-release preparations, particularly when used in doses of 2000 mg per day or more (JM McKenney et al, JAMA, 271:672, 1994).

FIBRIC ACID DERIVATIVES — **Gemfibrozil** *(Lopid)* lowers VLDL and can increase HDL cholesterol. It is also highly effective in lowering plasma triglycerides, but when the triglyceride concentration decreases, LDL cholesterol may increase in some patients. A five-year double-blind trial (the Helsinki Heart Study) in 4,081 asymptomatic hypercholesterolemic men showed not only decreased triglycerides, decreased LDL cholesterol and increased HDL cholesterol in men treated with gemfibrozil, but also a decrease in the number of myocardial infarctions from 84 with placebo to 56 with the drug. The decrease in infarctions occurred predominantly in a subgroup of patients with serum triglycerides higher than 200 mg/dl and a LDL/HDL cholesterol ratio greater than 5 (V Manninen et al, Circulation, 85:37, 1992). After an additional 3.5 years of follow-up in which more patients chose to take gemfibrozil, cardiovascular mortality was similar in the two groups originally assigned to gemfibrozil or placebo (OP Heinonen et al, J Intern Med, 235:41, 1994). In the Helsinki Heart Study and its follow-up, the incidence of gastrointestinal symptoms was slightly increased in men taking gemfibrozil, and cholecystectomies were more frequent, suggesting increased biliary cholesterol saturation, which may increase formation of cholesterol gallstones. Appendectomies were also more frequent in gemfibrozil-treated patients. Gemfibrozil may potentiate the effect of oral anticoagulants and oral hypoglycemic agents (*The Medical Letter Handbook of Adverse Drug Interactions*, 1995, p 152).

Clofibrate – Clofibrate (*Atromid-S*, and others) is a fibric acid derivative similar to gemfibrozil. Hypercholesterolemic men treated with clofibrate had an increased rate of mortality due to malignant and gastrointestinal disease, and a higher rate of cholecystectomy for gallstones (Committee of Principal Investigators, Br Heart J, 40:1069, 1978; JA Heady et al, Lancet, 340:1405, 1992). Use of the drug should be limited to patients with severe hypertriglyceridemia unresponsive to niacin and gemfibrozil.

PROBUCOL — Probucol *(Lorelco)* is relatively ineffective in lowering LDL and has the disadvantage of lowering HDL. The drug inhibits oxidation of LDL and decreases its uptake by macrophages, which theoretically could inhibit atherogenesis without decreasing serum cholesterol concentrations (D Steinberg and JL Witztum, JAMA, 264:3047, 1990).

FISH OIL — Large amounts of long-chain, highly unsaturated omega-3 fatty acids (present in cold water fish and commercially available in capsules) can decrease triglycerides and cause small decreases (or sometimes increases) in LDL cholesterol, without affecting HDL cholesterol (Medical Letter, 29:7, 1987). No studies are available comparing the effectiveness or safety of fish oil with other lipid-lowering drugs. Although a moderate intake of fish or alpha-linolenic acid (a precursor of omega-3 fatty acids) has had a favorable effect on mortality after myocardial infarction (ML Burr et al, Lancet, 2:757, 1989; M de Lorgeril et al, Lancet, 343:1454, 1994), it has not been possible to show a similar effect by increasing the intake of fish in men without cardiovascular disease (A Ascherio et al, N Engl J Med, 332:977, 1995). Omega-3 fatty acids from fish can interfere with platelet function, but bleeding has not been reported.

POSTMENOPAUSAL HORMONES — Postmenopausal treatment with estrogen alone or with progestins has been associated with substantial reductions in the risk of heart disease (D Grady et al, Ann Intern Med, 117:1016, 1992; BM Psaty et al, Arch Intern Med, 154:1333, 1994). In a placebo-controlled, three-year, double-blind study of 875 women with LDL cholesterol below 190 mg/dl and triglycerides below 500 mg/dl, estrogen alone or with a progestin lowered LDL and increased both triglycerides and HDL cholesterol compared to placebo (Writing Group for the PEPI Trial, JAMA, 273:199, 1995). Estrogen alone or combined with a progestin has also lowered plasma levels of lipoprotein(a) (CJ Kim et al, Arterioscler Thromb, 14:275, 1994).

Adverse Effects – Unopposed estrogen causes endometrial hyperplasia and increases the risk of endometrial cancer. Combined hormonal treatments using estrogen with a progestin do not. Whether estrogen alone or with a progestin could increase the risk of breast cancer is still unclear. One report suggested that postmenopausal hormone therapy was associated with an increased risk of systemic lupus erythematosus (J Sánchez-Guerrero et al, Ann Intern Med, 122:430, 1995).

COMBINATIONS — When tolerable doses of a single drug do not lower blood lipids sufficiently, two or even three drugs can be used together. Use of two drugs at relatively low dosage rather than a single drug at a high level may decrease adverse effects and cost less (HG Schrott et al, Am J Cardiol, 75:34, 1995). In patients with hypercholesterolemia, concurrent use of an HMG-CoA reductase inhibitor with a bile acid sequestrant or niacin effectively lowers LDL. For combined hypercholesterolemia and hypertriglyceridemia, concurrent use of an HMG-CoA reductase inhibitor with niacin may be helpful. In severe hypertriglyceridemia not adequately controlled by diet and a single drug, combining niacin with gemfibrozil may substantially lower triglyceride concentrations.

CONCLUSION — HMG-CoA reductase inhibitors are drugs of first choice for treatment of most patients with hypercholesterolemia. They are more effective and better tolerated than other cholesterol-lowering drugs and may slow the progression of coronary artery disease.

COST OF SOME CHOLESTEROL-LOWERING DRUGS

Drug	Daily dosage	Cost*
Cholestyramine – *Questran, Questran Light* (Bristol-Myers Squibb)	8 grams resin, divided	$ 49.70
Colestipol – *Colestid* (Upjohn)	10 grams, divided	44.64
Colestid tablets	8 grams, divided	68.76
Clofibrate – *Atromid S* (Wyeth-Ayerst)	1 gram bid	50.76
Fluvastatin – *Lescol* (Sandoz)	20 mg once**	31.92
Gemfibrozil – *Lopid* (Parke-Davis)	1200 mg, in 2 doses	65.74
Lovastatin – *Mevacor* (Merck)	20 mg once	62.53
Niacin – average generic price	1 gram tid	8.01
Niacor (Upsher-Smith)		24.20
Nicolar (Rhône-Poulenc Rorer)		115.92
Pravastatin – *Pravachol* (Bristol-Myers Squibb)	20 mg once	54.53
Probucol – *Lorelco* (Marion Merrell Dow)	500 mg bid	69.62
Simvastatin – *Zocor* (Merck)	10 mg once	56.39

* Cost to the pharmacist for 30 days' treatment based on wholesale price (AWP) listings in *Drug Topics Red Book*, 1995 and May *Update*.

** Dosage recommended by manufacturer but appears to be less potent than recommended doses of other HMG-CoA reductase inhibitors.

CHOICE OF CONTRACEPTIVES

New information about contraceptives continues to become available. The commonly used methods of reversible contraception are listed below.

METHODS OF CONTRACEPTION

Method and mechanism of action	Failure rate* Typical Use	Perfect Use	Some adverse effects or disadvantages	Some advantages
No method	85%			
Periodic abstinence Avoidance of coitus during presumed fertile days	20%			
Spermicide alone Inactivation of sperm	21%	6%	Vaginal irritation	May protect against some sexually transmitted diseases (STDs)
Cervical cap with spermicide Mechanical barrier; inactivation of sperm	18%	11.5%	Cervical irritation, may be difficult to fit, Pap smear abnormalities	Protection against STDs
Diaphragm with spermicide Mechanical barrier; inactivation of sperm	18%	6%	Cervical irritation, increased risk of urinary tract infection	Protection against STDs
Condom Mechanical barrier				
male	12%	3%	Allergic reactions	Protection against STDs
female	21%	5%	Difficult to insert, poor acceptability	Protection against STDs, including external genitalia

(continued)

Method and mechanism of action	Failure rate* Typical Use	Perfect Use	Some adverse effects or disadvantages	Some advantages
Oral contraceptives	3%			
Combined Suppression of ovulation, changes in cervical mucus and endometrium		0.1%	Rare thromboembolism and stroke, myocardial infarction in older smokers, nausea, headache, depression	Protection against ovarian and endometrial cancer, pelvic inflammatory disease, fibrocystic breast disease, ovarian cysts, iron-deficiency anemia and dysmenorrhea
Progestin only Changes in cervical mucus and endometrium, possibly suppression of ovulation		0.5%	Irregular, unpredictable bleeding in some	Protection against pelvic inflammatory disease, iron-deficiency anemia and dysmenorrhea
Intrauterine devices Progesterone T *(Progestasert)* Copper T 380A *(ParaGard)* Inhibition of sperm migration, fertilization and ovum transport	2% 0.8%	1.5% 0.6%	Increased ectopic pregnancy with progesterone device, rare uterine perforation, increase in menstrual blood loss with copper device	Decrease in menstrual blood loss and dysmenorrhea with progesterone device Copper device can be left in place for 10 years
Medroxyprogesterone acetate *(Depo-Provera)* Suppression of ovulation, changes in cervical mucus and endometrium	0.3%	0.3%	Menstrual irregularities, headache, weight gain, acne	Effective for 3 months
Levonorgestrel subdermal implants *(Norplant)* Similar to progestin only	0.09%	0.09%	Menstrual irregularities, headache, weight gain, acne, removal problems	Ease of use, reversibility, effective for 5 years

* Percent accidental pregnancy during first year of use, modified from RA Hatcher et al, *Contraceptive Technology*, 16th ed., New York:Irvington, 1994, page 113.

ORAL CONTRACEPTIVES — Oral contraceptives are usually a combination of an estrogen and a progestin. Taken conscientiously, they seldom fail, although some antibiotics and anticonvulsants taken concurrently can decrease their effectiveness (*The Medical Letter Handbook of Adverse Drug Interactions,* 1995, page 106). Biphasic and triphasic oral contraceptives vary the dosage of progestin and sometimes of estrogen in two or three phases, but have no demonstrated clinical advantage. Oral contraceptives containing only a progestin have a slightly higher failure rate and may cause irregular bleeding; their principal indications are for use during breast-feeding, for women who have contraindications to estrogens (such as hypertension or breast cancer) and for smokers more than 35 years old.

SOME ORAL CONTRACEPTIVES

Drug	Estrogen (μg)[1]	Progestin (mg)[2]	Cost[3]
COMBINATION			
Loestrin 1/20 21, 28 (Parke-Davis)	ethinyl estradiol (20)	norethindrone acetate (1)	$ 25.24
Loestrin 1.5/30 21, 28 (Parke-Davis)	ethinyl estradiol (30)	norethindrone acetate (1.5)	25.24
Levlen 21, 28 (Berlex)	ethinyl estradiol (30)	levonorgestrel (0.15)	21.15
Nordette-21 (Wyeth-Ayerst)[4]	ethinyl estradiol (30)	levonorgestrel (0.15)	21.03
Lo/Ovral (Wyeth-Ayerst)[4]	ethinyl estradiol (30)	norgestrel (0.3)	26.21
Desogen (Organon)	ethinyl estradiol (30)	desogestrel (0.15)	19.55
Ortho-Cept 21,28 (Ortho)[4]	ethinyl estradiol (30)	desogestrel (0.15)	22.20
Tri-Levlen 21, 28 (Berlex)	ethinyl estradiol (30, 40, 30)	levonorgestrel (0.05, 0.075, 0.125)	19.73
Triphasil-21 (Wyeth-Ayerst)[4]	ethinyl estradiol (30, 40, 30)	levonorgestrel (0.05, 0.075, 0.125)	25.03
Ortho Tri-Cyclen (Ortho)[4]	ethinyl estradiol (35, 35, 35)	norgestimate (0.18, 0.215, 0.25)	22.20
Ovcon 35 21, 28 (Bristol-Myers Squibb)	ethinyl estradiol (35)	norethindrone (0.4)	24.63

Drug	Estrogen (μg)[1]	Progestin (mg)[2]	Cost[3]
Brevicon 21, 28 (Syntex)	ethinyl estradiol (35)	norethindrone (0.5)	$ 22.94
Genora 0.5/35 28 (Rugby)	ethinyl estradiol (35)	norethindrone (0.5)	12.10
Modicon 21 (Ortho)[4]	ethinyl estradiol (35)	norethindrone (0.5)	25.36
Nelova 0.5/35 28 (Warner-Chilcott)	ethinyl estradiol (35)	norethindrone (0.5)	13.97
Tri-Norinyl 21,28 (Syntex)	ethinyl estradiol (35, 35, 35)	norethindrone (0.5, 1.0, 0.5)	21.38
Ortho-Novum 7/7/7 21 (Ortho)[4]	ethinyl estradiol (35, 35, 35)	norethindrone (0.5, 0.75, 1.0)	23.29
Nelova 10/11 28 (Warner-Chilcott)	ethinyl estradiol (35)	norethindrone (0.5, 1)	13.97
Ortho-Novum 10/11 21 (Ortho)[4]	ethinyl estradiol (35, 35)	norethindrone (0.5, 1.0)	25.36
Jenest-28 (Organon)	ethinyl estradiol (35)	norethindrone (1)	17.52
Genora 1/35 21, 28 (Rugby)	ethinyl estradiol (35)	norethindrone (1)	12.10
Nelova 1/35 21 (Warner-Chilcott)[4]	ethinyl estradiol (35)	norethindrone (1)	12.38
Norethin 1/35E 21, 28 (Roberts)	ethinyl estradiol (35)	norethindrone (1)	11.65
Norinyl 1/35 21, 28 (Syntex)	ethinyl estradiol (35)	norethindrone (1)	22.24
Ortho-Novum 1/35 21 (Ortho)[4]	ethinyl estradiol (35)	norethindrone (1)	23.14
Ortho-Cyclen (Ortho)[4]	ethinyl estradiol (35)	norgestimate (0.25)	22.20
Demulen 1/35 21 (Searle)[4]	ethinyl estradiol (35)	ethynodiol diacetate (1)	24.22
Genora 1/50 21, 28 (Rugby)	mestranol (50)	norethindrone (1)	12.10
Nelova 1/50 21 (Warner-Chilcott)[4]	mestranol (50)	norethindrone (1)	12.38
Norethin 1/50M 21, 28 (Roberts)	mestranol (50)	norethindrone (1)	11.65
Norinyl 1/50 21, 28 (Syntex)	mestranol (50)	norethindrone (1)	22.24
Ortho-Novum 1/50 21 (Ortho)[4]	mestranol (50)	norethindrone (1)	23.14

Drug	Estrogen (μg)[1]	Progestin (mg)[2]	Cost[3]
Ovral (Wyeth-Ayerst)[4]	ethinyl estradiol (50)	norgestrel (0.5)	$ 32.90
Ovcon 50 28 (Bristol-Myers Squibb)	ethinyl estradiol (50)	norethindrone (1)	27.18
Demulen 1/50 21 (Searle)[4]	ethinyl estradiol (50)	ethynodiol diacetate (1)	27.00
PROGESTIN ONLY			
Ovrette (Wyeth-Ayerst)	none	norgestrel (0.075)	21.90
Nor-QD (Syntex)	none	norethindrone (0.35)	27.09
Micronor (Ortho)	none	norethindrone (0.35)	29.22

1. Ethinyl estradiol and mestranol are not equivalent on a milligram basis; 35 μg of ethinyl estradiol are equivalent to 50 μg of mestranol.
2. Different progestins are not equivalent on a milligram basis.
3. Cost to the pharmacist for one month's use, based on wholesale price (AWP) listings in *Drug Topics Red Book* 1995 and May *Update.*
4. Also available in 28-day regimen at slightly different cost.

Safety – The most recent evidence suggests that the health benefits of combination oral contraceptives outweigh the risks. Women who have used various combination oral contraceptives, even for a short time, have had a lower incidence of endometrial and ovarian cancer (DA Grimes and KE Economy, Am J Obstet Gynecol, 172:227, 1995), while thromboembolic events associated with these agents have been rare. Whether the lower doses of estrogen in most current oral contraceptives offer an even lower risk of thromboembolic events or equal protection against endometrial and ovarian cancer is unclear (JW Goldzieher, Am J Obstet Gynecol, 171:587, 1994). Most studies have found no overall increase in the risk of breast cancer in women who have taken oral contraceptives, but the risk might be slightly increased in women less than 35 years old (PA Wingo et al, Obstet Gynecol, 78:161, 1991). Whether the newer progestins desogestrel and norgestimate cause fewer androgenic effects, such as acne, hirsutism and weight gain, than older progestins remains to be established (K Fotherby and ADS Caldwell, Contraception, 49:1, 1994).

Emergency Contraception – In high doses, some combination oral contraceptives taken after coitus can prevent fertilization or implantation of the fertilized ovum. *Ovral,* two tablets q12h x 2, or the lower-estrogen-dose contraceptives *Lo/Ovral, Nordette, Levlen,*

Triphasil (yellow pills only) or *Trilevlen* (yellow pills only), 4 tablets q12h x 2, begun within 72 hours after intercourse, can usually prevent pregnancy (Medical Letter, 37:9 and 36, 1995).

INTRAUTERINE DEVICES — Two intrauterine devices (IUDs) are currently marketed in the USA; both have a "T" shape and are medicated, one with progesterone and the other with copper. The *Progestasert* releases progesterone from the vertical stem of the T. It offers two important non-contraceptive advantages: less menstrual blood loss and less dysmenorrhea. A disadvantage is that the *Progestasert* must be replaced annually. The copper T380A (*ParaGard* – Medical Letter, 30:25, 1988) provides better contraceptive effectiveness and has remained effective for 10 years.

Contraindications to IUDs include nulliparity, mucopurulent cervicitis and recent pelvic inflammatory disease. The risk of pelvic inflammatory disease is increased with intrauterine devices, but the highest risk occurs in the first 20 days after insertion and the overall risk is minimal in women with no history of sexually transmitted diseases. Women who become pregnant with the *Progestasert* in place have an increased risk of ectopic pregnancy.

SPERMICIDES — Nonoxynol-9, the most commonly used spermicide in the USA, is a chemical surfactant that destroys the cell wall of sperm and may offer some protection against sexually transmitted diseases, including cervical cancer. With spermicidal foam, the container must be shaken thoroughly to disperse the spermicide before use. Spermicidal tablets or suppositories need 10 to 30 minutes to dissolve. A nonoxynol-9-containing polyvinyl alcohol film (*VCF* – Apothecus), which dissolves on insertion, must be placed in the vagina at least five minutes before intercourse, and its effectiveness is not well established. With all of these products, additional spermicide must be used each time intercourse is repeated. Spermicides can cause local irritation in either partner.

BARRIER DEVICES — Condoms for Men – Most condoms in the USA are made of latex, which is impermeable to viruses; a few are made from young lamb intestine, which is not. Latex can, however, cause allergic reactions in men or women, especially with continued exposure. Lotions or lubricants containing mineral oil can decrease the barrier strength of latex condoms by 90% in as little as 60 seconds (B Voeller et al, Contraception, 39:95, 1989); water-soluble lubricants are preferred. A polyurethane condom for men *(Avanti)*, which is nonallergenic and thinner than a latex condom, but may also break more frequently, is now available in some parts of the USA (Contraceptive Technology Update, 16 suppl, June 1995).

Condoms for Women – New condoms designed to be worn by women offer increased coverage of external genitalia and therefore, theoretically, increased protection against sexually transmitted diseases. The *Reality* vaginal pouch (Wisconsin Pharmacal) is a polyurethane sheath with a closed end that is inserted into the vagina while the open end rests outside on the labia (Medical Letter, 35:123, 1993).

Diaphragms – A diaphragm plus spermicide can be inserted as long as six hours before coitus. The device should be left in place for at least six hours after intercourse, but no longer than 24 hours. Additional spermicide is required for repeated intercourse.

Cervical cap – The *Prentif* cervical cap is a rubber device smaller than a diaphragm that fits over the cervix like a large thimble (Medical Letter, 30:93, 1988). The cap, which can be left in place for up to 48 hours, remains effective for more than one episode of intercourse without adding more spermicide. Some women cannot use the cap because of the limited number of sizes.

Sponges – The nonprescription vaginal contraceptive sponge containing one gram of nonoxynol-9 *(Today)* is moistened in water and inserted into the vagina near the cervix. Unlike spermicides used alone, the sponge can protect during multiple acts of coitus. The only manufacturer of sponges in the USA discontinued production in early 1995.

PERIODIC ABSTINENCE — Periodic abstinence refers to avoidance of intercourse during the presumed fertile times of the menstrual cycle. Four methods have generally been used: the calendar (rhythm), temperature, cervical mucus, and sympto-thermal, which is the most difficult, but also the most effective (DR Mishell, Jr, N Engl J Med, 320:777, 1989). Relatively long periods of abstinence are necessary with all four methods.

MEDROXYPROGESTERONE ACETATE — Injection of 150 mg of medroxyprogesterone acetate *(Depo-Provera)* intramuscularly every three months is a highly effective method of contraception. Irregular bleeding can be troublesome at first, but after one year of use most women are completely amenorrheic. In one study, bone density was lower in women who had used medroxyprogesterone acetate for five years, but in another it increased when the drug was discontinued (T Cundy et al, BMJ, 308:247, 1994).

PROGESTIN IMPLANTS — The *Norplant System* (Medical Letter, 33:17, 1991) requires subcutaneous implantation in the arm of six silicone rubber capsules containing levonorgestrel. The capsules release a small amount of the progestin into the circulation, providing highly effective contraception for five years, although they may become less effective in heavy women in the fourth and fifth years of use (Gu Su-Juan et al, Obstet Gynecol, 83:673, 1994). Both insertion and removal require local anesthesia, and in some women have been associated with skin damage and keloid formation (TJ Zuber et al, J Fam Pract, 34:613, 1992). These implants appear to be highly effective and safe. Their use by adolescents has been associated with high rates of continued use and low rates of pregnancy (M Polaneczky et al, N Engl J Med, 331:1201, 1994; VE Cullins et al, Obstet Gynecol, 83:1026, 1994).

DRUGS FOR EPILEPSY

Treatment of epilepsy should begin with a single drug, increasing the dosage gradually until seizures are controlled or adverse effects become intolerable. If seizures continue and further increases in dosage appear inadvisable because of adverse effects, at least one and sometimes a second alternative drug should be tried before considering use of two drugs at the same time. Most of the drugs used to treat epilepsy interact with each other and with other drugs; for details, see *The Medical Letter Handbook of Adverse Drug Interactions*, 1995. The treatment of status epilepticus is not included here.

CARBAMAZEPINE — Carbamazepine (*Tegretol*, and others), which is available only for oral use, is particularly effective for treatment of partial and secondarily generalized tonic-clonic seizures, but it can make absence or myoclonic seizures worse. Carbamazepine induces its own metabolism; serum concentrations often fall after a few weeks of treatment. Therapeutic failure associated with poor bioavailability has been reported with both generic carbamazepine and with *Tegretol*, particularly when tablets are stored in humid conditions.

Adverse Effects – Carbamazepine can cause rash, drowsiness, blurred vision, transient diplopia, headache, ataxia, nausea and vomiting, and it can interfere with cognitive function in learning situations. A mild leukopenia, which does not require stopping treatment, is fairly common. With high doses, reversible hypofibrinogenemia and thrombocytopenia can occur. Agranulocytosis, aplastic anemia, Stevens-Johnson syndrome, cardiac toxicity, hypo-osmolality due to an antidiuretic effect, aseptic meningitis, intractable diarrhea and hepatitis, which can be fatal, are rare. Circulating concentrations of thyroid hormones may be depressed, while TSH remains normal. Carbamazepine has been associated with neural tube defects in 1% of exposed pregnancies (FW Rosa, N Engl J Med, 324:674, 1991). Prophylactic use of folic acid may prevent or decrease the incidence of neural tube defects (AE Czeizel and I Dudas, N Engl J Med, 327:1832, 1992).

PHENYTOIN (diphenylhydantoin) — Phenytoin (*Dilantin*, and others), which is available for both oral and parenteral use, is as effective as carbamazepine for treatment of partial and secondarily generalized tonic-clonic seizures. Different formulations of phenytoin may not be equivalent to each other; dissolution problems have been reported with *Dilantin Kapseals*.

Adverse Effects – Nystagmus may occur with therapeutic serum concentrations of phenytoin and is nearly always present at higher concentrations. At serum concentrations higher than 20 µg/ml, drowsiness, ataxia and diplopia may occur. Gingival hyperplasia, coarsening of facial features and hirsutism can be troublesome. A morbilliform or scarlatiniform rash may occur, usually in the first 10 days of treatment, and rarely progresses to exfoliative dermatitis or the Stevens-Johnson syndrome. Phenytoin may interfere with cognitive function in learning situations. Less common adverse effects include megaloblastic anemia, a lupus-like syndrome, hepatic granulomas, hepatitis leading rarely to fatal hepatic necrosis, lymphadenopathy, peripheral neuropathy, nephritis, and rickets and osteomalacia due to increased vitamin D metabolism. Serum folic acid, thyroxine and vitamin K concentrations may decrease with long-term therapy, and bleeding disorders have been reported in infants born to mothers taking phenytoin. Fetal exposure to phenytoin has been associated with congenital anomalies, including oral cleft and cardiac abnormalities.

VALPROATE — Valproate, which is marketed as valproic acid (*Depakene*, and others) or divalproex sodium *(Depakote)*, is approved by the US Food and Drug Administration (FDA) only for treatment of absence seizures or multiple seizure types that include absence. Because it is effective and usually well tolerated, however, valproate is also widely used for generalized tonic-clonic, myoclonic and atonic seizures, especially for patients with more than one type of generalized seizures (R Davis et al, Drugs, 47:332, 1994; JM Pellock, Epilepsia, 35 suppl 4:S11, 1994). In one controlled trial, valproate was less effective than carbamazepine in controlling complex partial seizures, but equally effective for secondarily generalized seizures (RH Mattson et al, N Engl J Med, 327:765, 1992).

Adverse Effects – Drowsiness due to valproate is usually mild and transient, and adverse cognitive effects are minimal. Serious adverse effects of the drug are uncommon, but fatal liver failure has occurred, particularly in children less than two years old taking valproate in combination with other anticonvulsants; liver failure has also been reported in older children and adults taking valproate alone (St A. König et al, Epilepsia, 35:1005, 1994). Even in the absence of hepatic dysfunction, valproate can interfere with conversion of ammonia to urea and infrequently causes lethargy associated with increased blood ammonia concentrations (SK Kulick and DA Kramer, Ann Emerg Med, 22:610, 1993). Pancreatitis can occur (JJ Asconapé et al, Epilepsia, 34:177, 1993), and interstitial nephritis has been reported.

More common adverse effects of valproate include nausea and vomiting, which may be minimized by using the enteric-coated formulation (*Depakote*) or by taking the drug with food. Weight gain, transient hair loss, tremor and dose-related thrombocytopenia are also fairly common. Menstrual disturbances, polycystic ovaries and hyperandrogenism may occur with increased frequency in women taking valproate (JIT Isojärvi et al, N Engl J Med, 329:1383, 1993). Edema requiring diuretics for control has been reported. Congenital malformations have been associated with use of valproate during pregnancy, particularly with high plasma concentrations during the first trimester (D Battino et al, Acta Neurol Scand, 85:204, 1992; S Koch et al, Neurology, 42 suppl 5:83, 1992); neural tube defects appear to be the most common abnormality, occurring in 1.5% to 2% of exposed pregnancies (D Lindhout et al, Neurology, 42 suppl 5:94, 1992). Prophylactic use of folic acid may prevent or decrease the incidence of neural tube defects (AE Czeizel and I Dudas, N Engl J Med, 327:1832, 1992).

PHENOBARBITAL — Phenobarbital is an alternative drug for treatment of generalized tonic-clonic seizures and partial seizures. Its half-life is about 100 hours, and steady-state serum concentrations may not be reached for several weeks. Rapid absorption has made phenobarbital a common choice for seizures in infants, but adverse effects on cognitive function and school performance have led to decreased use in older children and adults. Sedation and behavior disturbances including hyperactivity, loss of concentration, and depression are the principal adverse effects. As with phenytoin and primidone, hemorrhage due to vitamin K deficiency can occur in infants born to mothers treated with phenobarbital. Like other anticonvulsants, barbiturates may be teratogenic.

PRIMIDONE — Primidone (*Mysoline*, and others) is effective for the same types of seizures as phenobarbital. The anticonvulsant effect is due both to the drug itself and its metabolites, which include phenobarbital; when monitoring is necessary, both primidone and phenobarbital concentrations should be measured. Sedation, vertigo, nausea and ataxia occur frequently unless the drug is started in very low dosage. Primidone can also cause disturbed behavior, difficulty concentrating and loss of libido.

ETHOSUXIMIDE — Ethosuximide *(Zarontin)* is recommended for treatment of uncomplicated absence seizures and is usually well tolerated. Adverse effects may include nausea, vomiting, lethargy, hiccups, headache and mood changes. Blood dyscrasias, erythema multiforme, Stevens-Johnson syndrome and a lupus-like syndrome have been reported. Psychotic behavior can occur with toxic serum concentrations.

FELBAMATE — Felbamate *(Felbatol)* was approved by the FDA for use alone or with other drugs in adults with partial and secondarily generalized seizures and as adjunctive therapy in children with the multiple types of seizures associated with the Lennox-Gastaut syndrome. A growing number of reports of aplastic anemia and acute hepatic failure have limited use of the drug.

GABAPENTIN — Gabapentin *(Neurontin)* has been approved for use as adjunctive therapy in adults and children over the age of 12 years with refractory partial and secondarily generalized seizures (Medical Letter, 36:39, 1994). Its role in treating other types of seizures remains to be determined. Gabapentin is not metabolized and is almost completely excreted by the kidneys. Unlike other antiepileptic drugs, gabapentin does not induce or inhibit hepatic microsomal enzymes and does not affect the metabolism of other antiepileptic drugs taken concurrently. Gabapentin also is generally well tolerated. Adverse effects, which include somnolence, dizziness, ataxia, fatigue and nystagmus, are usually mild and often transient. The drug's safety during pregnancy is unknown. Gabapentin has been associated with pancreatic acinar cell cancer in male rats receiving very high doses.

LAMOTRIGINE — Lamotrigine *(Lamictal)* is the newest antiepileptic drug marketed in the USA (Medical Letter, 37:21, 1995). Although approved in the USA only as adjunctive therapy for adults with uncontrolled partial seizures, addition of lamotrigine to other drugs may also be effective in idiopathic generalized seizures, including tonic-clonic and absence seizures and those associated with the Lennox-Gastaut syndrome. In two controlled trials in patients with newly diagnosed partial or generalized seizures, lamotrigine alone was as effective as carbamazepine or phenytoin, and better tolerated (MJ Brodie et al, Lancet, 345:476, 1995; TJ Steiner et al, Epilepsia, 35 suppl 7:61, 1994). The most common adverse effects of lamotrigine include rash, somnolence, blurred vision, dizziness, headache, diplopia, ataxia, nausea and vomiting. A rash occurs in about 10% of treated patients, usually in the first two weeks of drug administration. The rash usually disappears when the drug is stopped. A few patients have developed a severe rash, including Stevens-Johnson syndrome. The drug's safety in pregnancy is unknown.

CLONAZEPAM — Clonazepam *(Klonopin)* is a benzodiazepine used to treat myoclonic, atonic, and absence seizures that may be resistant to treatment with other anticonvulsants. It is generally less effective for absence seizures than ethosuximide or valproate, and development of tolerance to its effects is common. Adverse effects of clonazepam include drowsiness, drooling, ataxia and behavior disorders.

COST OF SOME ANTIEPILEPTIC DRUGS

Drug	Usual daily dosage	Cost*
Carbamazepine – average generic price	800 to 1600 mg	$ 28.19
Tegretol (Basel)		32.40
Clonazepam – *Klonopin* (Roche Labs)	1.5 to 20 mg	62.86
Ethosuximide – *Zarontin* (Parke-Davis)	750 to 1250 mg	64.55
Felbamate – *Felbatol* (Wallace)	1200 to 3600 mg	51.84
Gabapentin – *Neurontin* (Parke-Davis)	900 to 2400 mg	81.00
Lamotrigine – *Lamictal* (Burroughs Wellcome)	100 to 500 mg	49.80
Phenobarbital – average generic price	90 to 150 mg	.99
Phenytoin – average generic price	300 to 400 mg	5.40
Dilantin Kapseals (Parke-Davis)		16.26
Primidone – average generic price	750 to 1250 mg	32.04
Mysoline (Wyeth-Ayerst)		42.69
Valproate	1000 to 3000 mg	
Valproic acid – average generic price		39.97
Depakene (Abbott)		134.38
Divalproex sodium – *Depakote* (Abbott)		67.54

* Cost for 30 days' treatment with lowest recommended dosage, according to wholesale price (AWP) listings in *Drug Topics Red Book* 1995 and May *Update*.

TREATMENT OF SEIZURES

Seizure disorder		Drugs
PRIMARY GENERALIZED TONIC-CLONIC *(GRAND MAL)*		
	Drugs of Choice:	Valproate[2]
		OR Carbamazepine
		OR Phenytoin
	Alternatives:	Lamotrigine
		Primidone
		Phenobarbital
PARTIAL, INCLUDING SECONDARILY GENERALIZED		
	Drugs of Choice:	Carbamazepine
		OR Phenytoin
		OR Valproate[2]
	Alternatives:	Primidone
		Phenobarbital
		Lamotrigine (as adjunct)
		Gabapentin (as adjunct)
ABSENCE *(PETIT MAL)*		
	Drugs of Choice:	Ethosuximide
		OR Valproate
	Alternatives:	Clonazepam
		Lamotrigine
ATYPICAL ABSENCE, MYOCLONIC, ATONIC		
	Drug of Choice:	Valproate[2]
	Alternatives:	Clonazepam
		Felbamate (as adjunct)

1. Some patients obtain complete seizure control at lower concentrations, and occasional patients need higher concentrations. Serum concentrations may be altered by concurrent use of other drugs.
2. Not FDA-approved unless absence is involved.
3. Intolerance to carbamazepine can often be avoided by starting with 100 to 200 mg b.i.d. and increasing the dosage at weekly intervals in increments of 100 to 200 mg per day, up to the usual maintenance dosage.
4. Monitoring serum concentrations of carbamazepine alone may occasionally be misleading because the assay does not account for an active metabolite, carbamazepine-10,11 epoxide, which contributes to antiepileptic activity and also causes toxic effects. Serum measurements of the active metabolite are available but may be too expensive for routine use.

Usual daily dosage Adults	Children	Usual therapeutic serum concentrations[1]
1000-3000 mg	15-60 mg/kg	50-120 µg/ml
800-1600 mg[3]	10-30 mg/kg	6-12 µg/ml[4]
300-400 mg[5]	4-8 mg/kg	10-20 µg/ml
100-500 mg	Not approved	Not established
750-1250 mg	10-20 mg/kg	6-12 µg/ml
90-150 mg	2-5 mg/kg	15-35 µg/ml
800-1600 mg[3]	10-30 mg/kg	6-12 µg/ml[4]
300-400 mg[5]	4-8 mg/kg	10-20 µg/ml
1000-3000 mg	15-60 mg/kg	50-120 µg/ml
750-1250 mg[6]	10-20 mg/kg	6-12 µg/ml
90-150 mg	2-5 mg/kg	15-35 µg/ml
100-500 mg	Not approved	Not established
900-2400 mg[7]	Not approved	Not established
750-1250 mg	20-40 mg/kg	40-100 µg/ml
1000-3000 mg	15-60 mg/kg	50-120 µg/ml
1.5-20 mg	0.05-0.2 mg/kg	20-80 ng/ml
100-500 mg	Not approved	Not established
1000-3000 mg	15-60 mg/kg	50-120 µg/ml
1.5-20 mg	0.05-0.2 mg/kg	20-80 ng/ml
1200-3600 mg	15-60 mg/kg	Not established

5. Adjustments in dosage above 300 mg/day for adults should usually be made in 25 or 30 mg increments because of saturation kinetics.
6. Start with 50-100 mg daily and increase gradually at two- to three-day intervals.
7. Start with a dose of 300 mg once or twice daily and increase rapidly up to maintenance dosage.

DRUGS FOR CHRONIC HEART FAILURE

In recent years, cardiologists have emphasized the importance of neurohormonal as well as hemodynamic factors in the etiology of chronic heart failure (M Packer, Lancet, 340: 88, 92, 1992). Drugs that act on different factors are commonly used together.

ACE INHIBITORS — Angiotensin-converting enzyme (ACE) inhibitors interfere with formation of angiotensin II, an important vasoconstrictor in patients with heart failure. Although any ACE inhibitor might be effective for treatment of heart failure, captopril *(Capoten)* and enalapril *(Vasotec)* have been studied most extensively. Clinical trials have shown that ACE inhibitors improve symptoms and exercise tolerance in patients with heart failure, sometimes within days, but more commonly with a delay of four to twelve weeks. Controlled trials have also shown that these drugs slow the progression of heart failure and can prolong survival in patients with symptoms, and also in those with no symptoms but with impaired left ventricular function (SOLVD Investigators, N Engl J Med, 325:293, 1991; CONSENSUS Trial Study Group, N Engl J Med, 316:1429, 1987; MA Pfeffer et al for SAVE Investigators, N Engl J Med, 327:669, 1992; SOLVD Investigators, N Engl J Med, 327:685, 1992). The optimal dosage of ACE inhibitors needed to achieve these effects remains undefined; most controlled clinical trials used captopril 50 mg t.i.d. or enalapril 10 mg b.i.d.

The most common adverse effects of ACE inhibitors are cough, hypotension and renal insufficiency; decreasing the dosage of diuretics taken concurrently may ameliorate hypotension and renal insufficiency. ACE inhibitors may also cause rash, taste disturbances and angioedema.

DIURETICS — Most patients with heart failure have fluid retention and require diuretics. By decreasing fluid retention, diuretics relieve symptoms in patients with chronic heart failure and may prevent clinical deterioration but, given alone, their effect on clinical deterioration is weak and their effect on survival is unknown. The diuretic most commonly used in the USA for treatment of heart failure is furosemide (*Lasix*, and others), usually in an initial dose of 20 to 40 mg orally. Diuretics that act on the loop of Henle, such as furosemide, bumetanide *(Bumex)* or torsemide (*Demadex* – Medical Letter, 36:73, 1994), are more effective for treatment of heart failure than thiazide diuretics, such as chlorothiazide (*Diuril*, and others), which act on the distal tubule. Patients resistant to an oral diuretic may respond to intravenous administration or to concurrent use of two diuretics with different mechanisms of action. Nonsteroidal anti-inflammatory drugs decrease renal blood flow and decrease the response to diuretic drugs. Excessive doses of diuretics should be avoided especially in patients also taking an ACE inhibitor, because volume depletion may lead to ACE inhibitor toxicity (DW Baker et al, JAMA, 272:1361, 1994).

The most common adverse effect of diuretic therapy is potassium depletion, which can be decreased or avoided by concurrent use of a potassium-sparing diuretic such as spironolactone (*Aldactone*, and others), amiloride (*Midamor*, and others) or triamterene (*Dyrenium*), or an ACE inhibitor. Using both a potassium-sparing diuretic and an ACE inhibitor can produce dangerous degrees of hyperkalemia. Magnesium depletion can also occur with diuretics; amiloride, but not spironolactone, may have magnesium-sparing properties (DL Murdoch et al, Br J Clin Pharmacol, 35:373, 1993). In patients with renal dysfunction, diuretics may cause azotemia.

DIGITALIS — Despite more than 200 years of use, the effectiveness of digitalis glycosides in treating heart failure has only recently been demonstrated in controlled trials. Two placebo-controlled trials in a total of 266 patients treated for mild to moderate chronic heart failure found that when digoxin (*Lanoxin*, and others) was withdrawn, exercise capacity was more likely to decrease and symptoms of heart failure were more likely to become worse than when placebo was withdrawn, whether or not the patients were also taking an ACE inhibitor (BF Uretsky et al for PROVED Investigators, J Am Coll Cardiol, 22:955, 1993; M Packer et al for

RADIANCE Investigators, N Engl J Med, 329:1, 1993). The clinical benefits of digoxin may be due to its positive inotropic effect and/or to suppression of the increased sympathetic activity characteristic of chronic heart failure (H Krum et al, J Am Coll Cardiol, 25:289, 1995). The effect of digoxin on the survival of patients with heart failure is still unknown.

The optimal dosage of digoxin is not clear. Clinical studies have often used a daily dosage of 0.25 to 0.50 mg, but many clinicians prescribe 0.125 to 0.25 mg daily. Since serum concentrations as low as 0.4 ng/ml of digoxin may be effective, determination of digoxin concentrations should be used primarily to identify toxicity; concentrations of less than 2.0 ng/ml are usually well tolerated. The most common adverse effects of digitalis glycosides are cardiac arrhythmias, conduction disturbances, neurological disturbances and gastrointestinal symptoms. Hypokalemia or renal insufficiency markedly increases the risk of toxicity.

HYDRALAZINE-NITRATE COMBINATION — The combination of hydralazine (*Apresoline*, and others), which dilates primarily arterial resistance vessels, and isosorbide dinitrate (*Isordil*, and others), which dilates primarily venous capacitance vessels, decreases both preload and afterload in the failing heart. In patients receiving digitalis and diuretics, addition of relatively large doses of isosorbide dinitrate (40 mg q.i.d.) and hydralazine (75 mg q.i.d.) increased left ventricular ejection fraction and decreased mortality, compared to placebo (JN Cohn et al for V-HeFT I Investigators, N Engl J Med, 314:1547, 1986); a subsequent trial found, however, that addition of an ACE inhibitor to digitalis and a diuretic had a more beneficial effect on mortality (JN Cohn et al for V-HeFT II Investigators, N Engl J Med, 325:303, 1991). Adverse effects, especially headache and gastrointestinal disturbances, occurred frequently with the combination of hydralazine and isosorbide dinitrate. The effectiveness and safety of hydralazine and isosorbide dinitrate in patients also taking an ACE inhibitor are unknown.

BETA-BLOCKERS — Beta-blockers have not been used in the past in patients with heart failure because they decrease contractility. The ability of these drugs to block the deleterious effects of the sympathetic nervous system can, however, benefit some patients with chronic heart failure (EJ Eichhorn, Am J Med, 92:527, 1992). The results of some controlled trials suggest that these drugs can improve symptoms and left ventricular function in patients with heart failure, particularly those with nonischemic dilated cardiomyopathy (F Waagstein et al, Lancet, 342:1441, 1993; CIBIS Investigators and Committees, Circulation, 90:1765, 1994). The long-term safety of these drugs for treatment of heart failure has not been established.

AMIODARONE — Patients with both heart failure and ventricular arrhythmias may benefit from fairly low doses of amiodarone (300 mg/day). One report suggested that such doses, which are not proarrhythmic and do not worsen left ventricular function, may decrease mortality (HC Doval et al, Lancet, 344:493, 1994). This study needs confirmation.

CONCLUSION — Patients with heart failure due to left ventricular dysfunction should take an ACE inhibitor, and most also require a diuretic to relieve congestion. Digitalis may benefit those who remain symptomatic after treatment with an ACE inhibitor and a diuretic. Patients who do not respond to or cannot tolerate an ACE inhibitor may benefit from a combination of hydralazine and isosorbide dinitrate.

DRUGS FOR HYPERTENSION

Drugs available in the USA for treatment of chronic hypertension, their dosages and adverse effects are listed in the table below and discussed in the text beginning on page 101. Drugs for treatment of hypertensive emergencies are not discussed here.

ORAL ANTIHYPERTENSIVE DRUGS

Drug and daily adult dosage	Cost[1]	Frequent or severe adverse effects
ANGIOTENSIN-CONVERTING ENZYME (ACE) INHIBITORS		
Benazepril – *Lotensin* 10-40 mg in 1 or 2 doses	$19.09	Cough; hypotension, particularly with a diuretic or volume depletion; loss of taste; rash; acute renal failure with bilateral renal artery stenosis or stenosis of the artery to a solitary kidney; angioedema; hyperkalemia if also taking potassium supplements or potassium-sparing diuretics; blood dyscrasias and renal damage rare except in patients with renal dysfunction; increased fetal mortality; may decrease excretion of lithium
Captopril – *Capoten* 12.5-150 mg in 2 or 3 doses	19.35[2]	
Enalapril – *Vasotec* 2.5-40 mg in 1 or 2 doses	21.53	
Fosinopril – *Monopril* 10-40 mg in 1 or 2 doses	21.26	
Lisinopril – *Prinivil* 5-40 mg in 1 dose	23.59	
Zestril	23.59	
Quinapril – *Accupril* 5-80 mg in 1 or 2 doses	27.27	
Ramipril – *Altace* 1.25-20 mg in 1 or 2 doses	17.72	
ANGIOTENSIN RECEPTOR ANTAGONIST		
Losartan – *Cozaar* 25-100 mg in 1 or 2 doses	$33.00[3]	Little experience, but apparently does not cause cough

1. Cost to the pharmacist for 30 days' treatment with the lowest recommended dosage, based on wholesale price (AWP) listings in *Drug Topics Red Book* 1995 and May *Update*.
2. Cost based on purchase of 30 of smallest tablet size available.
3. Wholesale price (AWP) listing in *First DataBank PriceAlert*, May 15, 1995

Drug and daily adult dosage	Cost[1]	Frequent or severe adverse effects
BETA-ADRENERGIC BLOCKING DRUGS		
Atenolol – 25-100 mg in 1 or 2 doses		Fatigue; depression; bradycardia; decreased exercise tolerance; congestive heart failure; aggravate peripheral arterial insufficiency; aggravate allergic reactions; bronchospasm; mask symptoms of and delay recovery from hypoglycemia; Raynaud's phenomenon; insomnia; vivid dreams or hallucinations; acute mental disorder; impotence; increased serum triglycerides, decreased HDL cholesterol; generalized pustular psoriasis; sudden withdrawal can lead to exacerbation of angina and myocardial infarction
average generic price	$20.26	
Tenormin	26.52	
Betaxolol – *Kerlone*	21.61[2]	
5-40 mg in 1 dose		
Bisoprolol – *Zebeta*	26.59	
5-20 mg in 1 dose		
Metoprolol – 50-200 mg in 1 or 2 doses		
average generic price	13.53	
Lopressor	15.62	
Toprol XL	13.39	
Nadolol – 20-240 mg in 1 dose		
average generic price	22.55	
Corgard	28.46	
Propranolol – 40-240 mg in 2 doses		
average generic price	4.10	
Inderal	18.77	
extended release – 80-240 mg in 1 dose		
average generic price	23.18	
Inderal-LA	26.91	
Timolol – 10-40 mg in 2 doses		
average generic price	16.97	
Blocadren	24.85	
BETA-ADRENERGIC BLOCKING DRUGS WITH INTRINSIC SYMPATHOMIMETIC ACTIVITY		
Acebutolol – *Sectral*	$28.08	Similar to other beta-adrenergic blocking drugs, but with less resting bradycardia and lipid changes; acebutolol has been associated with a positive antinuclear antibody test and occasional drug-induced lupus
200-1200 mg in 1 or 2 doses		
Carteolol – *Cartrol*	28.51	
2.5-10 mg in 1 dose		
Penbutolol – *Levatol*	29.20	
20-80 mg in 1 dose		
Pindolol – 10-60 mg in 2 doses		
average generic price	36.64	
Visken	46.12	

(continued)

Drug and daily adult dosage	Cost[1]	Frequent or severe adverse effects
ALPHA-BETA-BLOCKER		
Labetalol – 200-1200 mg in 2 doses		Similar to other beta-adrenergic blocking drugs, but has intrinsic sympathomimetic activity and more orthostatic hypotension; fever; hepatotoxicity
Normodyne	$25.52	
Trandate	25.52	
CALCIUM-CHANNEL BLOCKERS		
Diltiazem – extended-release		Dizziness; headache; edema; constipation (especially verapamil); AV block; bradycardia; heart failure; gingival hyperplasia
Cardizem SR	$48.00	
120-360 mg in 2 doses		
Cardizem CD	31.32	
120-360 mg in 1 dose		
Dilacor XR	27.79	
120-480 mg in 1 dose		
Verapamil – 20-480 mg in 2 or 3 doses		
average generic price	24.61	
Calan	29.85	
Isoptin	27.67	
extended-release[4] – 120-480 mg in 1 or 2 doses		
Calan SR	26.72	
Isoptin SR	26.72	
Verelan – 120-480 mg in 1 dose	32.30	
DIHYDROPYRIDINES		
Amlodipine – *Norvasc*	35.36	Dizziness; headache; peripheral edema (more than with verapamil and diltiazem); flushing; tachycardia; rash; gingival hyperplasia
2.5-10 mg in 1 dose		
Felodipine – *Plendil*	25.62	
5-20 mg in 1 dose		
Isradipine – *DynaCirc*	23.71	
5-10 mg in 1 or 2 doses		
Nicardipine – *Cardene*	36.64	
60-120 mg in 3 doses		
extended-release – 60-120 mg in 2 doses		
Cardene SR	38.15	
Nifedipine – extended-release		
30-90 mg in 1 dose		
Adalat CC	26.11	
Procardia XL	36.96	

4. Available generically in 180- or 240-mg extended-release tablets.

Drug and daily adult dosage	Cost[1]	Frequent or severe adverse effects
DIURETICS		
THIAZIDE-TYPE (Usually once daily)		
Bendroflumethiazide – *Naturetin* 2.5-5 mg	$23.18[2]	Hyperuricemia; hypokalemia; hypomagnesemia; hyperglycemia; hyponatremia; hypercalcemia; hypercholesterolemia; hypertriglyceridemia; pancreatitis; rashes and other allergic reactions; sexual dysfunction; photosensitivity reactions; may decrease excretion of lithium
Benzthiazide – *Exna* 12.5-50 mg	5.99[2]	
Chlorothiazide – 125-500 mg		
average generic price	1.82[2]	
Diuril	3.92[2]	
Hydrochlorothiazide – 12.5-50 mg		
average generic price	1.04[2]	
Esidrix	3.61[2]	
Hydroflumethiazide – 12.5-50 mg		
Saluron	15.91[2]	
Diucardin	13.69[2]	
Methyclothiazide – 2.5-5 mg		
average generic price	2.45[2]	
Enduron	11.97[2]	
Polythiazide – *Renese* 1-4 mg	12.37	
Trichlormethiazide – 1-4 mg		
average generic price	2.87[2]	
Naqua	10.70[2]	
Metahydrin	12.76[2]	
Chlorthalidone – 12.5-50 mg		
average generic price	2.27[2]	
Hygroton	19.74[2]	
Indapamide – *Lozol* 2.5-5 mg	25.42	
Metolazone		
Zaroxolyn – 1.25-5 mg	12.86[2]	
Mykrox – 0.5-1 mg	21.24	

(continued)

Drug and daily adult dosage	Cost[1]	Frequent or severe adverse effects
LOOP		
Bumetanide – *Bumex*	$ 8.80[2]	Dehydration; circulatory collapse; hypokalemia; hyponatremia; hypomagnesemia; hyperglycemia; metabolic alkalosis; hyperuricemia; blood dyscrasias; rashes; lipid changes as with thiazide-type diuretics
0.5-5 mg in 2 or 3 doses		
Furosemide		
20-320 mg in 2 doses		
average generic price	1.73[2]	
Lasix	4.73[2]	
Torsemide – *Demadex*	13.13	
5-20 mg in 1 or 2 doses		
POTASSIUM-SPARING		
Amiloride – *Midamor*	$13.40[2]	Hyperkalemia; GI disturbances; rash; headache
5-10 mg in 1 or 2 doses		
Spironolactone		Hyperkalemia; hyponatremia; mastodynia; gynecomastia; menstrual abnormalities; GI disturbances; rash
12.5-100 mg in 1 or 2 doses		
average generic price	2.51[2]	
Aldactone	11.59[2]	
Triamterene – *Dyrenium*	9.77	Hyperkalemia; GI disturbances; nephrolithiasis
50-150 mg in 1 or 2 doses		
SOME COMBINATIONS		
Hydrochlorothiazide 25 mg-spironolactone 25 mg (50 mg-50 mg)		
1 tablet in 1 dose		
– average generic price	$ 2.42	
Aldactazide	12.49	
Hydrochlorothiazide 25 mg-triamterene 37.5 mg (25 mg-50 mg; 50 mg-75 mg)		
1-2 capsules in 1 dose		
– generic price (Geneva)	10.33	Similar to individual components
Dyazide	12.03	
½-1 tablet in 1 dose		
– average generic price	9.38[2]	
Maxzide	12.38[2]	
Hydrochlorothiazide 50 mg-amiloride 5 mg		
½-1 tablet in 1 dose		
– average generic price	9.81[2]	
Moduretic	15.62[2]	

Drug and daily adult dosage	Cost[1]	Frequent or severe adverse effects
ALPHA-ADRENERGIC BLOCKERS		
Prazosin		Syncope with first dose; dizziness and vertigo; palpitations; fluid retention; headache; drowsiness; weakness; anticholinergic effects
First day: 1 mg at bedtime		
Maintenance: 1-20 mg in 2 doses		
average generic price	$ 7.72[2]	
Minipress	12.43[2]	
Terazosin – *Hytrin*	36.67	Similar to prazosin
First day: 1 mg at bedtime		
Maintenance: 1-20 mg in 1 dose		
Doxazosin – *Cardura*	26.60	Similar to prazosin, but with less hypotension after first dose
First day: 1 mg at bedtime		
Maintenance: 1-16 mg in 1 dose		
CENTRAL SYMPATHOLYTICS		
Clonidine		CNS reactions similar to methyldopa, but more sedation and dry mouth; bradycardia; heart block; rebound hypertension (less likely with patches); contact dermatitis from patches
0.1-0.6 mg in 2 doses		
average generic price	$ 2.54[2]	
Catapres	16.85[2]	
transdermal – *Catapres TTS*	29.19	
one patch weekly		
(0.1 to 0.3 mg/day)		
Guanabenz – *Wytensin*		
4-64 mg in 2 doses	21.05[2]	Similar to clonidine
Guanfacine – *Tenex*	24.91	Similar to clonidine, but milder
1-3 mg in 1 dose		
Methyldopa		Drowsiness; sedation; fatigue; depression; dry mouth; orthostatic hypotension; bradycardia; heart block; autoimmune disorders, including colitis; hepatitis; hepatic necrosis; Coombs' positive hemolytic anemia; lupus-like syndrome; thrombocytopenia; red cell aplasia
250 mg-2 grams in 2 doses		
average generic price	6.94	
Aldomet	16.13	

Drug and daily adult dosage	Cost[1]	Frequent or severe adverse effects
DIRECT VASODILATORS		
Hydralazine		Tachycardia; aggravation of angina; headache; dizziness; fluid retention; nasal congestion; lupus-like syndrome; hepatitis
40-200 mg in 2 to 4 doses		
average generic price	$ 4.61	
Apresoline	24.72	
Minoxidil		Tachycardia; aggravation of angina; marked fluid retention; possible pericardial effusion; hair growth on face and body
2.5-40 mg in 1 or 2 doses		
average generic price	8.91	
Loniten	11.94	
PERIPHERAL ADRENERGIC NEURON ANTAGONISTS		
Guanethidine – *Ismelin* 10-100 mg in 1 dose	$14.90	Orthostatic hypotension; exercise hypotension; diarrhea; bradycardia; sodium and water retention; retrograde ejaculation
Guanadrel – *Hylorel* 10-75 mg in 2 doses	21.60[2]	Similar to guanethidine, but less diarrhea
Reserpine – 0.05-0.1 mg in 1 dose		Psychic depression; nightmares; nasal stuffiness; drowsiness; GI disturbances; bradycardia
average generic price	1.17[2]	

Trade Names	Components
COMBINATIONS	
BETA-ADRENERGIC BLOCKERS AND DIURETICS	
Corzide	nadolol 40 or 80 mg bendroflumethiazide 5 mg
*Inderide**	propranolol 40 or 80 mg hydrochlorothiazide 25mg
Inderide LA	propranolol 80, 120 or 160 mg hydrochlorothiazide 50 mg
Lopressor HCT	metoprolol 50 or 100 mg hydrochlorothiazide 25 or 50 mg
*Tenoretic**	atenolol 50 or 100 mg chlorothalidone 25 mg
Timolide	timolol 10 mg hydrochlorothiazide 25 mg
Ziac	bisoprolol 2.5, 5 or 10 mg hydrochlorothiazide 6.25 mg

(continued)

Trade Names	Components
ACE INHIBITORS AND DIURETICS	
Capozide	captopril 25 or 50 mg hydrochlorothiazide 15 or 25 mg
Lotensin HCT	benazepril 5, 10, 20 mg hydrochlorothiazide 6.25, 12.5 or 25 mg
Prinzide	lisinopril 10 or 20 mg hydrochlorothiazide 12.5 or 25 mg
Vaseretic	enalapril 10 mg hydrochlorothiazide 25 mg
Zestoretic	lisinopril 20 mg hydrochlorothiazide 12.5 or 25 mg
ANGIOTENSIN II RECEPTOR ANTAGONIST AND DIURETIC	
Hyzaar	losartan 50 mg hydrochlorothiazide 12.5 mg
OTHER COMBINATIONS	
*Aldoril**	methyldopa 250 or 500 mg hydrochlorothiazide 15, 25, 30 or 50 mg
Apresazide	hydralazine 25 mg hydrochlorothiazide 25 mg
Esimil	guanethidine 10 mg hydrochlorothiazide 25 mg
*Hydropres**	reserpine 0.125 mg hydrochlorothiazide 25 or 50 mg

* Also available generically

ANGIOTENSIN-CONVERTING ENZYME (ACE) INHIBITORS — Ace inhibitors are effective and well tolerated for treatment of hypertension. They are less effective, but not necessarily ineffective, in black patients. ACE inhibitors have no adverse effects on plasma lipid concentrations or on glucose tolerance, and some have been shown to prolong survival in patients with heart failure or left ventricular dysfunction after a myocardial infarction (Medical Letter, 35:41, 1993; 36:69, 1994) and to preserve renal function in patients with diabetes (EJ Lewis et al, N Engl J Med, 329:1456, 1993; M Ravid et al, Ann Intern Med, 118:577, 1993).

Patients with high levels of plasma renin activity may have excessive hypotensive responses to ACE inhibitors; such patients include those who are volume-depleted or taking diuretics, and those with renovascular hypertension or congestive heart failure.

Patients with bilateral renovascular disease whose renal perfusion is being maintained by high levels of angiotensin II may develop acute renal failure when an ACE inhibitor is used. Cough occurs commonly in patients treated with these drugs (D Ravid et al, J Clin Pharmacol, 34:1116, 1994). One recent report suggests that inhalation of cromolyn *(Intal)* may relieve the cough (MR Hargreaves and MK Benson, Lancet, 345:13, 1995). Hyperkalemia can occur, particularly in patients taking potassium supplements or potassium-sparing diuretics, or those with decreased renal function. Angioedema, which may be life-threatening, occurs in 0.1% to 0.2% of patients. ACE inhibitors should not be used during pregnancy because of the risk of fetal injury and death (A Shotan et al, Am J Med, 96:451, 1994).

AN ANGIOTENSIN RECEPTOR ANTAGONIST — Losartan, a newly released drug that interferes with binding of angiotensin II to AT-1 receptors, might prove to be as effective as an ACE inhibitor, without causing a cough. Like ACE inhibitors, losartan may be less effective in black patients.

BETA-ADRENERGIC BLOCKING DRUGS — Beta-blockers are effective for treatment of hypertension, but like ACE inhibitors, may be somewhat less effective in black patients (BJ Materson et al, N Engl J Med, 328:914, 1993). In controlled trials, beta-blockers have been shown to decrease mortality in patients with hypertension and in patients who have had a myocardial infarction. Although they generally have not been recommended for patients with congestive heart failure, recent data suggest that beta-blockers may be beneficial in such patients when given in low initial doses and carefully monitored (EJ Eichhorn and A Hjalmarson, Circulation, 90:2153, 1994).

Propranolol, **timolol**, **nadolol**, **pindolol**, **penbutolol**, and **carteolol** are "nonselective" beta-blockers; **metoprolol**, **acebutolol**, **atenolol**, **betaxolol** and **bisoprolol** in low doses are "cardioselective," with a greater effect on cardiac ($beta_1$) adrenoreceptors than on $beta_2$-adrenergic receptors of the bronchi and blood vessels. Selectivity is an advantage for diabetic patients because selective beta-blockers are less likely to delay recovery from hypoglycemia or cause severe hypertension when hypoglycemia leads to an increase in circulating epinephrine. These drugs become less selective, however, as dosage is increased, and even low doses can cause bronchospasm in patients with asthma.

Pindolol, acebutolol, penbutolol, and **carteolol** have intrinsic sympathomimetic activity. Unlike other beta-blockers, they apparently do not increase serum triglyceride concentrations or decrease HDL cholesterol. In addition, they can lower blood pressure with less decrease in heart rate at rest and may be preferred for patients who develop symptomatic bradycardia with other beta-blockers. They have not, however, been shown to lower mortality after a myocardial infarction.

Labetalol combines nonselective beta-blockade with alpha-adrenergic receptor blockade. It decreases blood pressure more promptly than other beta-blockers, is equally effective in black and white patients and does not affect serum lipids. Orthostatic hypotension is more frequent than with other beta-blockers.

CALCIUM-CHANNEL BLOCKERS — The calcium-channel blockers cause vasodilatation, which decreases peripheral resistance. The cardiac response to the decrease in vascular resistance is variable; with some dihydropyridines (felodipine, isradipine, nicardipine, nifedipine), an initial reflex increase in heart rate usually occurs, but verapamil, diltiazem and amlodipine cause little or no change in heart rate. Verapamil and diltiazem can, however, affect atrioventricular (AV) conduction and should be used with caution in patients also taking a beta-blocker. Calcium-channel blockers, with the possible exception of amlodipine (Medical Letter, 34:99, 1992), should be used with caution in patients with heart failure or myocardial dysfunction. Unlike diuretics and beta-blockers, calcium-channel blockers do not affect serum lipid concentrations. One retrospective study in patients with hypertension, published to date only as an abstract, found use of calcium-channel blockers associated with an increased incidence of myocardial infarction (BM Psaty et al, Circulation, 91:925, 1995).

DIURETICS — Diuretics, like beta-blockers, have been shown to decrease mortality in patients with hypertension. Many

thiazide-type diuretics are used to treat hypertension; **hydrochlorothiazide** and **chlorthalidone** are the most widely used. **Metolazone** and **indapamide** (Medical Letter, 31:103, 1989) may be effective in patients with impaired renal function when thiazides are not. Many patients, particularly older ones, can be treated with small doses of diuretics equivalent to 12.5 mg to 25 mg of hydrochlorothiazide once daily. Doses as low as 6.25 mg are now used to enhance the effectiveness of other drugs while minimizing adverse effects. One study found that use of diuretics for hypertension was associated with an increased risk of sudden death, but not when doses were low or a potassium-sparing diuretic was added (DS Siscovick et al, N Engl J Med, 330:1852, 1994).

Loop diuretics can be used to treat hypertension in patients with renal insufficiency (serum creatinine above 1.5 mg/dl). In patients without renal insufficiency, loop diuretics are no more effective than thiazides for treatment of hypertension.

Potassium-sparing diuretics are used with other diuretics to prevent or correct hypokalemia. These drugs can cause hyperkalemia, particularly in patients with renal impairment and those taking other drugs that decrease aldosterone secretion, such as ACE inhibitors.

ALPHA-ADRENERGIC BLOCKING DRUGS — Alpha-blockers useful in treating hypertension act at vascular postsynaptic alpha receptors to produce arterial and venous dilatation. **Prazosin, terazosin** and **doxazosin** cause less tachycardia than direct vasodilators (hydralazine, minoxidil) but more frequent postural hypotension, particularly following the first dose of any of these drugs. In contrast to diuretics and beta-blockers, alpha-blockers do not adversely affect blood lipids; they may increase the HDL/total cholesterol ratio (BL Kasiske et al, Ann Intern Med, 122:133, 1995). Alpha-blockers may provide symptomatic relief from prostatism in men (Medical Letter, 36:15, 1994; JE Oesterling, N Engl J Med, 332:99, 1995), but they may also cause stress incontinence in women (PL Dwyer and JS Teele, Obstet Gynecol, 79:117, 1992), and the incidence of postural hypotension is higher in elderly patients.

CENTRAL SYMPATHOLYTICS — Drugs such as **clonidine**, **guanabenz**, **guanfacine** and **methyldopa** do not inhibit reflex responses as completely as sympatholytic drugs that act peripherally, but frequently cause sedation, dry mouth and depression.

DIRECT VASODILATORS — Direct vasodilators frequently produce reflex tachycardia, and rarely cause orthostatic hypotension. They should usually be given with a beta-blocker or a centrally-acting drug to minimize the reflex increase in heart rate and cardiac output, and with a diuretic to avoid sodium and water retention. With **hydralazine**, maintenance dosage should be limited to 200 mg per day to decrease the possibility of a lupus-like reaction. **Minoxidil**, a potent drug that rarely fails to lower blood pressure, should be reserved for severe hypertension refractory to other drugs. Minoxidil usually causes hirsutism and can cause severe fluid retention.

PERIPHERAL ADRENERGIC NEURON ANTAGONISTS — These drugs can cause troublesome adverse effects and are seldom used now. **Reserpine** is an inexpensive and effective antihypertensive drug (FA Lederle et al, Arch Intern Med, 153:705, 1993); given in doses higher than now recommended, it can cause severe depression. **Guanethidine** usually decreases cardiac output and may lower systolic pressure more than diastolic; postural and exertional hypotension occur commonly and are aggravated by vasodilatation caused by a hot environment, exercise or alcohol. **Guanadrel** is similar to guanethidine, with a much shorter duration of action.

COMBINATION PRODUCTS — Thiazide diuretics are available in fixed-dose combinations with potassium-sparing diuretics and with other antihypertensive drugs. Combination products are convenient, but many Medical Letter consultants prefer to adjust the dosage of each drug separately. When the optimum maintenance doses correspond to the ratio in a combination product, taking fewer tablets may improve compliance.

INTERACTIONS — In addition to the adverse effects listed in the table, antihypertensive drugs may interact adversely with other drugs taken at the same time (*The Medical Letter Handbook of Adverse Drug Interactions*, 1995). One particularly important interaction can occur with nonsteroidal anti-inflammatory drugs (NSAIDs), which can decrease the effectiveness of many antihypertensive agents (AG Johnson et al, Ann Intern Med, 121:289, 1994).

CHOICE OF DRUGS — All the drugs approved for treatment of hypertension in the USA are effective in lowering blood pressure. Diuretics, beta-adrenergic blockers, ACE inhibitors and calcium-channel blockers are the best tolerated. Only diuretics and beta-blockers have been shown in large-scale clinical trials to decrease mortality in patients with hypertension. ACE inhibitors, calcium-channel blockers and alpha-adrenergic blockers have, however, a more favorable effect on some cardiovascular risk factors.

In special categories of patients, one drug may offer advantages over the others. Diuretics and calcium-channel blockers are more effective than beta-blockers or ACE inhibitors in **black patients**. Patients with **diabetes**, particularly with nephropathy, may benefit most from an ACE inhibitor. For patients with **hyperlipidemia**, an ACE inhibitor, alpha-blocker or calcium-channel blocker might be a good choice. Patients with **congestive heart failure** may gain extra benefit from an ACE inhibitor. A beta-blocker (without intrinsic sympathomimetic activity) may be indicated for hypertensive patients with **angina pectoris** or **migraine**, and for those who have had a **myocardial infarction**.

Even when drugs are carefully chosen to fit individual needs, patients' responses may vary (S Attwood et al, J Hypertension, 12:1053, 1994). If the first drug chosen is ineffective or poorly tolerated, a drug from another class should be substituted. If more than one drug is necessary and a diuretic was not used initially, most Medical Letter consultlants would add a diuretic.

DRUGS FOR MIGRAINE

Drugs are used both to prevent and treat migraine symptoms. The effectiveness of such use can be difficult to evaluate, even with double-blind controlled trials, because migraine is episodic, response to placebo is frequent, and patients vary in response to a given agent (KMA Welch, N Engl J Med, 329:1476, 1993; SD Silberstein and RB Lipton, Neurology, 44 suppl 7:S6, 1994).

SOME DRUGS FOR TREATMENT OF MIGRAINE

Drug	Dosage[1]	Cost[2]
Acetaminophen 325 mg - isometheptene 65 mg - dichloralphenazone 100 mg	2 capsules, then 1 q1h PRN (max. 5 q12h)	
average generic price		$ .93
Midrin (Carnrick)		1.85
Aspirin 325 mg - caffeine 40 mg - butalbital 50 mg	1 to 2 tablets or capsules q4h (max. 6 q24h)	
average generic price - tablets		.44
average generic price - capsules		2.19
Fiorinal (Sandoz)		2.87
Butorphanol	One spray in one nostril; can be repeated once in 3 to 5 hrs	
Stadol NS (Bristol-Myers Squibb)		7.66 to 14.36[3]
Dihydroergotamine	1 mg IM; can be repeated twice at 1-hour intervals	
D.H.E. 45 (Sandoz)		30.81

(continued)

1. Recommended by the manufacturer.
2. Cost of treating one migraine attack using highest recommended dosage based on wholesale price (AWP) listings in *Drug Topics Red Book* 1995 and May *Update*.
3. Each 2.5 ml bottle contains 25 mg of butorphanol and supplies 8 to 15 1-mg doses depending on frequency of use.

Drug	Dosage[1]	Cost[2]
Ergotamine 1 mg - caffeine 100 mg	2 tablets orally, then 1 q30min. x 4 PRN (max. 6 mg/attack)	
average generic price		2.95
Ergotamine 2 mg - caffeine 100 mg	One rectal suppository; can be repeated once in one hour	
average generic price		5.30
Cafergot (Sandoz)		7.88
Sumatriptan – *Imitrex* (Cerenex)	6 mg subcutaneously	35.34

TREATMENT — Analgesics – Treatment with any one of various analgesics may be sufficient for mild or moderate forms of migraine. **Aspirin** can be effective; it is widely used for treatment of migraine both alone and in combinations such as *Fiorinal* (aspirin, caffeine, butalbital). **Acetaminophen** has been used for migraine both alone and in combinations such as *Midrin* with isometheptene, a mild sympathomimetic, and dichloralphenazone, a sedative. **Nonsteroidal anti-inflammatory drugs (NSAIDs)** have also been effective in relieving the pain of some migraine attacks. In one study, naproxen sodium *(Anaprox)* was at least as effective as ergotamine tartrate in aborting acute headache in 79 patients with migraine (TA Treves et al, Headache, 32:280, 1992). Decreased gastric motility during an acute migraine attack may interfere with absorption of analgesics, and over-frequent use (daily or almost daily) of analgesic combinations can cause an increase in headache ("analgesic rebound"). **Metoclopramide** (*Reglan*, and others) may enhance the absorption of aspirin and other oral medications by increasing gastric motility and may prevent the nausea associated with many migraine attacks, especially if begun promptly at the onset of symptoms. Rarely, however, it can cause an acute dystonic reaction. A double-blind controlled trial in 96 patients with migraine found that **butorphanol** nasal spray *(Stadol NS)*, an opioid agonist-antagonist, was more effective than placebo or intramuscular methadone *(Dolophine)* for relief of moderate to severe migraine headache pain (S Diamond et al, Headache Quarterly, 3:164, 1992). Opioid adverse effects such as drowsiness may be troublesome, however, and psychiatric reactions have occurred (Medical Letter, 35:105, 1993).

Ergotamine tartrate, a serotonin agonist, has been widely used for treatment of moderate to severe migraine headaches (B Baumel, Neurology, 44 suppl 3:S13, 1994); it is most effective when taken early in an attack but may still be effective even if treatment is delayed. When used more than two days in a week, it can cause dependence (rebound headache). Manufacturers of ergot products have had some production problems recently; ergotamine is now available only in combinations. Nausea and vomiting are fairly common with ergotamine, but can be prevented by concurrent use of an antiemetic. Serious adverse effects, including vascular occlusion and gangrene, are rare but can occur with overdosage (more than 6 mg in 24 hours or 10 mg per week). These effects may be potentiated by beta-adrenergic blockers, dopamine (*Intropin*, and others), erythromycins or troleandomycin *(Tao)* (*The Medical Letter Handbook of Adverse Drug Interactions*, 1995, page 138). Liver disease or fever can accelerate symptoms of ergotism.

Dihydroergotamine *(D.H.E. 45)*, a derivative of ergotamine, can be injected subcutaneously, intramuscularly or intravenously and will soon be available in an intranasal spray (Dihydroergotamine Nasal Spray Multicenter Investigators, Headache, 35:177 1995). Like ergotamine, it has been effective in treating acute attacks of migraine unresponsive to analgesics (AK Scott, Clin Neuropharmacol, 15:289, 1992). Dihydroergotamine is a much weaker vasoconstrictor than ergotamine and causes fewer adverse effects; it can cause diarrhea and muscle cramps, but dependence (rebound headache) apparently does not occur.

Sumatriptan *(Imitrex)* has been marketed in the USA in a formulation designed for patients to inject themselves subcutaneously; an oral formulation, already available in Europe and Canada, will probably be marketed here soon. A nasal spray, commercially available in some countries, is being used experimentally in the USA (R Salonen et al, J Neurol, 241:463, 1994). A serotonin agonist with a short duration of action, it appears to be more effective than ergotamine for treatment of acute migraine attacks, but no controlled clinical trial comparing the two has been published (Medical Letter, 34:91, 1992). One double-blind, placebo-controlled trial in 171 patients found that giving sumatriptan subcutaneously during a migraine aura before the onset of headache had no effect on the duration of the aura and did not delay or prevent development of headache (D Bates et al, Neurology, 44:1587, 1994).

Tingling, flushing, burning of the skin at the site of injection, a general feeling of heaviness and a sense of tightness and pressure in the chest may occur with the injectable preparation. Angina has been reported with both the injectable and oral preparation in patients with coronary artery disease. One patient who injected herself with 6-mg doses of sumatriptan subcutaneously for cluster headache had chest pain after the first and second injections one day apart and, with a third injection one week later, developed an acute myocardial infarction (JP Ottervanger et al, Lancet, 341:861, 1993). Current labeling for the drug states that it "...should not be given to patients in whom unrecognized coronary artery disease (CAD) is likely without a prior evaluation for underlying cardiovascular disease. Such patients include postmenopausal women, males over 40, and patients with risk factors for CAD such as hypertension, hypercholesterolemia, obesity, diabetes, smokers, and strong family history..." Chest discomfort after sumatriptan is usually benign, however, and may sometimes be esophageal in origin (LA Houghton et al, Lancet, 344:985, 1994).

The oral dosage of sumatriptan in Canada is one 100-mg tablet. The subcutaneous dosage is one 6-mg injection, given preferably in the lateral thigh or deltoid. A second dose has not usually been effective if pain does not respond to the first, but is recommended for treatment of a recurrent migraine attack. The maximum dosage in a 24-hour period is three tablets or two injections; injections should be separated by at least one hour. Sumatriptan should not be used within 24 hours after use of any ergotamine-containing drug because vasoconstriction could be additive, and patients should be warned not to take ergot derivatives until six hours or more after sumatriptan.

Dihydroergotamine vs. Sumatriptan – An unpublished multicenter controlled trial compared a single subcutaneous injection of dihydroergotamine with sumatriptan for abortive treatment of moderate to severe migraine in 295 patients. After two hours 73%

of patients had relief with dihydroergotamine and 85% with sumatriptan, a statistically significant difference. By four hours, however, the percentage of patients relieved was about the same with either drug (85% vs. 83%), and at 24 hours 90% of patients treated with dihydroergotamine had relief, compared to 77% with sumatriptan. Headache recurred in the 24 hours after treatment in 18% of patients treated with dihydroergotamine and 45% treated with sumatriptan (R Ricalder et al, Presented at the Annual Meeting of the American Academy of Family Physicians, Sept 1994, Boston).

SOME DRUGS FOR PREVENTION OF MIGRAINE

Drug	Dosage[1]	Cost[2]
Methysergide – *Sansert* (Sandoz)	2 to 4 mg b.i.d.	$ 98.53
Propranolol	40 to 120 mg b.i.d.	
average generic price		6.20
Inderal (Wyeth-Ayerst)		24.86
Timolol	10 to 15 mg b.i.d.	
average generic price		20.34
Blocadren (Merck)		30.73

1. Recommended by the manufacturer.
2. Cost to the pharmacist for 30 days' treatment with lowest daily dosage based on wholesale price (AWP) listings in *Drug Topics Red Book* 1995 and May *Update*.

PROPHYLAXIS — Patients with frequent or severe migraine headaches or those refractory to symptomatic treatment may require prophylaxis. Menstrual or other predictable migraine attacks may sometimes be prevented by a brief course of ergotamine or an NSAID, such as naproxen, taken for several days before and during the first few days of menstruation (G Sances et al, Headache, 30:705, 1990).

For continuous prophylaxis, **beta-adrenergic blocking agents** are the most commonly used drugs. Propranolol (*Inderal*, and others) and timolol (*Blocadren*, and others) are the only beta-blockers approved by the US Food and Drug Administration for this indication. The dosage of propranolol recommended for migraine prophylaxis is 80 to 240 mg/day, but some patients benefit from and can tolerate higher doses; sustained-release *Inderal LA* can be taken in a single daily dose (KA Halroyd et al, Headache, 31:333,

1991). Timolol is usually given in a dosage of 10 mg twice daily, but can be taken in a single 20-mg dose. Nadolol *(Corgard)* and metoprolol (*Lopressor*, and others) have also been effective in preventing migraine, according to Medical Letter consultants. Some other beta-blockers, particularly those with intrinsic sympathomimetic activity (ISA), have been ineffective for migraine prophylaxis. All beta-blockers can cause fatigue, depression, orthostatic hypotension and other adverse effects; all are contraindicated in patients with asthma or congestive heart failure.

Methysergide *(Sansert)*, another ergot alkaloid, is effective for prevention of migraine, but may cause weight gain, peripheral edema and retroperitoneal, pleuropericardial and subendocardial fibrosis with prolonged (more than six months) use. Major vessel constriction, mesenteric vascular fibrosis and small bowel infarction have been reported rarely. Concurrent use with other ergot alkaloids, beta-adrenergic blockers, erythromycins, dopamine or troleandomycin may increase the risk of arterial spasm and occlusion (*The Medical Letter Handbook of Adverse Drug Interactions*, 1995, page 186). Methysergide should be reserved for recurrent, refractory severe migraine; many clinicians recommend an interval without the drug for four weeks every six months, but whether this practice decreases toxicity is unclear.

Calcium-channel blockers have also been tried for prophylaxis. Verapamil (*Calan, Isoptin*, and others) has been moderately effective in a few placebo-controlled trials (GD Solomon, Headache, 29:425, 1989), but nifedipine (*Procardia*, and others) has had mixed results in both abortive and prophylactic use (K-E Andersson and E Vinge, Drugs, 39:355, 1990; MJ Hoffert et al, Cephalalgia, 12:323, 1992). Flunarizine *(Sibelium)*, available in Canada but not in the USA, was at least as effective as propranolol or metoprolol in decreasing the number of attacks (MJ Gawel et al, Can J Neurol Sci, 19:340, 1992; P Soelberg Sørensen et al, Headache, 31:650, 1991). No calcium-channel blocker has been approved by the FDA for prevention of migraine.

Nonsteroidal anti-inflammatory drugs (NSAIDs), particularly naproxen sodium, have been used for prevention of migraine as well as for aborting acute attacks; the effectiveness of this practice is not well established. One study in 22,000 men found that 325 mg of **aspirin** every other day decreased the frequency of migraine headache by 20% (JE Buring et al, JAMA, 264: 1711, 1990).

Antidepressants can prevent migraine in some patients and may be given concurrently with other prophylactic agents. Amitriptyline (*Elavil*, and others), a tricyclic, in dosage ranging from 10 to 200 mg per day has probably been used more for this purpose than other antidepressants (DK Ziegler et al, Arch Neurol, 50:825, 1993). Whether fluoxetine *(Prozac)* or the other selective serotonin reuptake inhibitors (SSRIs) could be helpful for this indication remains to be established.

Valproate (divalproex – *Depakote*; valproic acid – *Depakene*, and others), an anticonvulsant also used for treatment of bipolar disorder (Medical Letter, 36:74, 1994), in dosage ranging from 800 to 1500 mg per day has been effective in preventing migraine in a few controlled trials (R Hering and A Kuritzky, Cephalalgia, 12:81, 1992; R Jensen et al, Neurology, 44:647, 1994; NT Mathew et al, Arch Neurol, 52:281, 1995).

CONCLUSION — An analgesic may be effective for treatment of mild or moderate migraine. Either sumatriptan or dihydroergotamine is the drug of choice for treatment of severe migraine headache; although currently available only for parenteral use, sumatriptan oral tablets and dihydroergotamine nasal spray may both be marketed here soon. A beta-blocker is the best established choice for prevention of migraine attacks.

DRUGS FOR PAIN

Three types of analgesic drugs are available in the USA: first, non-opioids, including aspirin, other nonsteroidal anti-inflammatory drugs (NSAIDs), and acetaminophen; second, opioids; and third, some drugs not usually thought of as analgesics, which act as adjuvants when given with NSAIDs or opioids, or have analgesic activity of their own in some types of pain (American Pain Society, *Principles of Analgesic Use*, 3rd ed, Skokie, Illinois:American Pain Society, 1992).

NSAIDs AND ACETAMINOPHEN — With increasing doses, aspirin, acetaminophen and the newer NSAIDs all reach a ceiling for their maximum analgesic effect. For aspirin and acetaminophen, the maximum analgesic effect usually occurs with doses between 650 and 1300 mg. The ceiling effect for some newer NSAIDs is relatively higher and the duration of analgesic effect may be longer than with aspirin or acetaminophen. With all of these drugs, patients evidently do not develop tolerance to their analgesic effects.

Aspirin – Controlled clinical trials have shown aspirin to be effective in most types of pain, including cancer pain. Inhibition of cyclooxygenase is probably the mechanism of aspirin's analgesic action and also the cause of most of its adverse effects. A single therapeutic dose irreversibly inhibits platelet function for the seven-day lifetime of the platelet, inhibiting hemostasis and prolonging bleeding time. A single dose of aspirin can also precipitate asthma in aspirin-sensitive patients. Multiple doses can cause gastropathy and salicylism.

Acetaminophen – Acetaminophen is as effective as aspirin, similar in potency and, in single analgesic doses, has the same time-effect curve, but does not have the adverse effects characteristic of aspirin. Large overdosage with acetaminophen can cause serious or fatal hepatic injury, and some patients, such as alcoholics, patients who are fasting and those taking cytochrome P-450 enzyme-inducing drugs concurrently, may develop hepatic injury after moderate overdosage. Most patients, however, can take 4 grams a day with no adverse effects (DC Whitcomb and GD Block, JAMA, 272:1845, 1994).

Other NSAIDs – In single full doses, most of the NSAIDs listed in the table on page 121 are more effective analgesics than full doses of aspirin or acetaminophen, and some can equal or exceed the analgesic effect of oral narcotic combination products, or even injected opioids. Whether this is also true with repeated doses in chronic pain is less well established, and few controlled trials comparing the newer NSAIDs with each other have been published. Some patients may respond better to one NSAID than another (WT Beaver in GM Aronoff ed, *Evaluation and Treatment of Chronic Pain*, 2nd ed., Baltimore:Williams & Wilkins, 1992, page 369).

Combinations – Aspirin, acetaminophen or NSAIDs can be given concurrently with opioids for an additive analgesic effect. Even when insufficient alone to control pain adequately, NSAIDs have an additive effect that permits use of lower dosage of opioids (CA Moote, Can J Anaesth, 41:527, 1994). There is no evidence that NSAIDs have additive effects when used with each other.

Adverse Effects of NSAIDs – The adverse effects of all NSAIDs are qualitatively similar to those of aspirin. Except for the risk of precipitating asthma and anaphylactoid reactions in aspirin-sensitive patients, single or a few doses of the newer oral NSAIDs cause few adverse effects. Unlike aspirin, NSAIDs cause reversible inhibition of platelet aggregation; platelet function returns when most of the drug has been eliminated.

With chronic use, upper gastrointestinal bleeding, ulceration and perforation can occur, sometimes without warning. There is some evidence from epidemiologic studies that ibuprofen in doses of 1600 mg/day or less causes less gastrointestinal toxicity than aspirin or other NSAIDs, but fatal hemorrhage and perforation have occurred with all of these drugs. High doses, a long half-life, prolonged use and advanced age are risk factors.

NSAIDs decrease synthesis of renal vasodilator prostaglandins, decrease renal blood flow, cause fluid retention, and may cause renal failure in some patients; risk factors include old age, congestive heart failure, chronic renal insufficiency, ascites, intravascular volume depletion and concurrent diuretic therapy. Rarely, NSAIDs cause allergic interstitial nephritis and the nephrotic syndrome, both usually reversible on discontinuation of the drug. Concurrent use of an NSAID decreases the effectiveness of many antihypertensive drugs (*Medical Letter Handbook of Adverse Drug Interactions*, 1995, page 208.)

Unlike opioids, NSAIDs have no potential for abuse. Physical dependence on these drugs has not been reported.

Ketorolac – Ketorolac is the only injectable NSAID available for analgesic use in the USA (Medical Letter, 32:79, 1990). Other parenteral NSAIDs have been marketed in other parts of the world, but adverse reactions at the site of injection have limited their usefulness. Intramuscular (IM) ketorolac is relatively nonirritating to tissues. The dose of IM or IV ketorolac should be reduced for patients more than 65 years old, for those weighing less than 50 kg and for patients with moderately elevated serum creatinine. Even with parenteral administration, gastric toxicity can occur. The combined duration of use of parenteral and oral ketorolac should not exceed 5 days. In one study, a single dose of ketorolac IV interfered with hemostasis after tonsillectomy in children (LM Rusy et al, Anesth Analg, 80:226, 1995).

OPIOIDS — Although considered the drugs of choice for severe acute pain and chronic cancer pain, the effectiveness of opioids overlaps with that of the NSAIDs. Oral codeine, its congeners, propoxyphene and pentazocine in usual doses are no more effective when taken alone than is aspirin or acetaminophen and are usually prescribed in combinations with these drugs to treat moderate or moderately severe pain. Morphine, hydromorphone, methadone, levorphanol, fentanyl and large doses of oxycodone are used for the most severe pain (KM Foley, N Engl J Med, 313:84, 1985). Opioids produce analgesia by binding to various opioid receptors within, and possibly outside, the central nervous system; they are classified as full agonists, partial agonists and mixed agonist-antagonists. Morphine and the other full agonists, unlike NSAIDs, have no ceiling for their analgesic effectiveness, except that imposed by adverse effects.

Choice of Opioid – While the parenteral full agonists listed in the table on page 124 differ in potency, they are all, with the exception of codeine, equally capable of relieving acute pain in the non-tolerant patient if the dose is adjusted appropriately.

Morphine – Morphine is generally considered the standard of comparison for strong injectable analgesics. Given orally, it is well absorbed but extensively metabolized on the first pass through the liver and has a short duration of action. Sustained-release oral preparations have a longer duration of action. The drug can also be given rectally. Morphine has no greater dependence liability than do equally effective doses of any full agonist.

Meperidine – Given intramuscularly, meperidine is irritating to tissues and short acting. Repeated doses of the drug lead to accumulation of normeperidine, a toxic metabolite with a 15- to 20-hour half-life that can cause dysphoria, irritability, tremors, myoclonus and, occasionally, seizures, particularly with large repeated doses or decreased renal function. In patients taking a monoamine oxidase inhibitor, meperidine can cause severe encephalopathy and death (*Medical Letter Handbook of Adverse Drug Interactions*, 1995, page 197).

Methadone and Levorphanol – Both of these drugs are sometimes used orally to relieve pain in patients with cancer, particularly those tolerant to morphine. Since, however, the average plasma half-life of methadone is 24 hours and that of levorphanol is 12 to 16 hours, repeated doses of either drug can lead to accumulation and central-nervous-system (CNS) depression, particularly in elderly or debilitated patients.

Tramadol – A new opioid agonist that also blocks norepinephrine and serotonin, tramadol is marketed for treatment of mild to moderate pain. Its effectiveness is comparable to that of codeine (CR Lee et al, Drugs, 46:313, 1993; A Sunshine, Drugs, 47 suppl 1:8, 1994).

Partial Agonists and Mixed Agonist-Antagonists – The partial agonist buprenorphine is similar to the mixed agonist/antagonists pentazocine, butorphanol, nalbuphine and dezocine. All of these drugs can precipitate withdrawal symptoms in patients physically dependent on full agonists. All are less likely to cause dependence than full agonists, but none is completely free of dependence liability. Only pentazocine is available for oral use and only in combination products.

Tolerance to Opioids – Tolerance is common with chronic use of opioids; the patient first notices a shorter duration of analgesia and then an increase in pain. Tolerance can be delayed by giving nonopioid analgesics concurrently. Tolerance to most of the adverse effects of opioids, including respiratory and CNS depression, develops at least as rapidly as tolerance to the analgesic effect. Tolerance, therefore, can usually be surmounted and adequate analgesia restored by increasing the dose. Cross-tolerance exists among all of the full agonists, but it is not complete, and switching to another opioid, starting with half the equianalgesic dose, may be helpful.

Dependence – Patients who take strong opioids will develop physical dependence and abstinence symptoms if the drug is discontinued suddenly or an opioid antagonist is given. Physical dependence can be detected after a few days of therapy, but clinically significant dependence develops only after several weeks of chronic treatment with relatively large doses of morphine-like opioids. Patients who take opioids for acute pain or cancer pain rarely experience euphoria and even more rarely develop psychological dependence or addiction to the mood-altering effects of narcotics (A Jacox et al, N Engl J Med, 330:651, 1994; A Jacox et al, *Clinical Practice Guideline*, No. 9, Rockville, MD:Agency for Health Care Policy and Research, 1994 [AHCPR publication no.94-0592]).

Adverse Effects – Sedation, grogginess, dizziness, nausea, vomiting and constipation are the most common adverse effects of opioids; respiratory depression is the most serious. Sedation can be ameliorated by decreasing the dose and increasing the frequency of administration, by switching to opioids with a shorter half-life, and by giving small oral doses of dextroamphetamine or methylphenidate (*Ritalin*, and others) in the morning and early afternoon (E Bruera et al, Pain, 50:75, 1992). Tolerance usually develops rapidly to the sedative and emetic effect of these drugs, but not to constipation.

In patients with chronic obstructive pulmonary disease, cor pulmonale, decreased respiratory reserve or pre-existing respiratory depression, even usual doses of opioids may decrease respiratory drive and cause apnea. Patients without pulmonary disease who take opioids chronically are often tolerant to the respiratory depressant effect, but the addition of general anesthetics, phenothiazines, tranquilizers, sedative-hypnotics, tricyclic antidepressants or other CNS depressants increases the risk.

Dosage – Opioid dose requirements may vary widely from one patient to another. For the nontolerant patient, the usual dose must frequently be increased to achieve adequate analgesia and occasionally decreased to avoid adverse effects. For most strong opioids, the dose should be increased until adverse effects occur before switching to another opioid. Once the optimal dose that will provide adequate analgesia, hopefully for at least four hours, has been established by titration, it should be given on a schedule, with the provision that the patient can refuse a dose if not in pain. "By-the-clock" administration of analgesics is much more effective than waiting for severe pain to return before giving the next dose and may decrease total dosage. An order for a supplementary opioid dose between regular doses, which may be the same or different from the regular medication, should be available as a rescue for breakthrough pain.

ADJUVANT ANALGESICS — Tricyclic antidepressants, such as amitriptyline (*Elavil*, and others), in doses lower than those used to treat depression can relieve many types of neuropathic pain, including post-herpetic neuralgia and diabetic neuropathy (MB Max et al, N Engl J Med, 326:1250, 1992). The anticonvulsants **carba-**

mazepine (*Tegretol*, and others), **clonazepam** (*Klonopin*) or **phenytoin** (*Dilantin*, and others) can relieve lancinating pain from trigeminal neuralgia, post-herpetic neuralgia, glossopharyngeal neuralgia and neuralgias arising from nerve trauma or infiltration with cancer (M Swerdlow, Clin Neuropharmacol, 7:51, 1984; RK Portenoy in D Doyle et al, eds, *The Oxford Textbook of Palliative Medicine*, Oxford:Oxford University Press, 1993, page 187).

Caffeine, although not an analgesic when given alone, in doses of 65 to 200 mg has been shown in controlled trials to enhance the analgesic effect of acetaminophen, aspirin or ibuprofen in headache, oral surgery pain and postpartum pain (EM Laska et al, JAMA, 251:1711, 1984; JA Forbes et al, Clin Pharmacol Ther, 49:674, 1991; JR Migliardi et al, Clin Pharmacol Ther, 56:576, 1994). **Hydroxyzine** (*Vistaril*, and others) in doses of 50 to 100 mg IM adds significantly to the analgesic effect of opioids in postoperative and cancer pain while reducing the incidence of nausea and vomiting.

Corticosteroids – Through their anti-inflammatory effect, corticosteroids can produce analgesia in some patients with inflammatory diseases or tumor infiltration of nerves (TA Rummans, Mayo Clin Proc, 69:481, 1994).

ACETAMINOPHEN AND NSAID ANALGESICS

Drug	Usual single analgesic dose	Dose interval	Maximum daily dose	Comments
Acetaminophen (*Tylenol*, others)	PO: 500-1000 mg	q4-6h	4000 mg	As effective as aspirin; 1000 mg usually more effective than 650 mg; duration of action usually 4 hours
Salicylates				
Aspirin (many manufacturers)	PO: 500-1000 mg	q4-6h	4000 mg	Duration of action after single doses usually 4 hours; active metabolite accumulates with repeated doses
Choline magnesium trisalicylate (*Trilisate*)	PO: 1000-1500 mg	q8-12h	3000 mg	Effectiveness compared to aspirin not clear; onset of analgesia probably slower; less gastropathy and impairment of platelet function
Diflunisal (*Dolobid*, and others)	PO: 1000 mg initial then 500 mg	q8-12h	1500 mg	500 mg superior to 650 mg of aspirin or acetaminophen, with slower onset and longer duration; comparable to acetaminophen/codeine combination
Other NSAIDs				
Diclofenac potassium (*Cataflam*)	PO: 50 mg	q8h	150 mg	Comparable to aspirin with longer duration
Etodolac (*Lodine*)	PO: 200-400 mg	q6-8h	1200 mg	Efficacy data limited; 200 mg comparable and 400 mg possibly superior to 650 mg of aspirin
Fenoprofen (*Nalfon*)	PO: 200 mg	q4-6h	1200 mg	Comparable to aspirin; contraindicated with impaired renal function

Drug	Usual single analgesic dose	Dose interval	Maximum daily dose	Comments
Flurbiprofen *(Ansaid)*	PO: 50-100 mg	q6-8h	300 mg	Analgesic indication not FDA-approved; 50 mg superior to 650 mg of aspirin with longer duration of action; 100 mg superior to acetaminophen/codeine combination
Ibuprofen *(Motrin, Rufen, Advil, Nuprin,* others)	PO: 200-400 mg	q4-8h	2400 mg	200 mg equal to 650 mg of aspirin and acetaminophen; 400 mg superior with longer duration; 400 mg comparable to acetaminophen/ codeine combination
Ketoprofen *(Orudis,* and others)	PO: 25-75 mg	q4-8h	300 mg	25 mg comparable to ibuprofen 400 mg and superior to 650 mg of aspirin; 50 mg superior to acetaminophen/ codeine combination
Ketorolac *(Toradol)*	IM: 60 mg as a single dose			Comparable to 12 mg IM morphine or 100 mg IM meperidine with longer duration; use should be limited to 5 days.
	Patients <65 y.o. IM or IV: 30 mg	q6h	120 mg	
	Patients ≥65 y.o. IM or IV: 15 mg	q6h	60 mg	
	PO: 10 mg	q6h	40 mg	10 mg superior to aspirin or acetaminophen or acetaminophen/codeine combination and comparable to ibuprofen 400 mg; combined parenteral and oral use should be limited to 5 days.
Meclofenamate *(Meclomen)*	PO: 50-100 mg	q4-8h	400 mg	Comparable to aspirin; approved for dysmenorrhea

Drug	Usual single analgesic dose	Dose interval	Maximum daily dose	Comments
Mefenamic acid *(Ponstel)*	PO: 500 mg initial then 250 mg	q6h	1250 mg	Comparable to aspirin but more effective in dysmenorrhea; duration of use not to exceed 1 week
Naproxen *(Naprosyn,* and others)	PO: 500 mg initial then 250 mg	q6-12h	1250 mg	250 mg probably comparable to 650 mg of aspirin with slower onset and longer duration; 500 mg superior to 650 mg of aspirin
Naproxen sodium *(Anaprox,* and others)	PO: 550 mg initial then 275 mg	q6-12h	1375 mg	275 mg comparable to 650 mg of aspirin with slower onset and longer duration; 550 mg superior to 650 mg of aspirin with comparable onset

OPIOID ANALGESICS

Drug	IM dose[1]	IM duration (hours)[2]	Starting oral dose[3]	Comments
Agonists related to morphine				
Morphine (*Duramorph*, and others)	10 mg	3-6	20-60 mg	Available as 8-12h sustained release tablets *(MS-Contin, Oramorph-SR)*
Hydromorphone *(Dilaudid)*	1.3 mg	3-5	4-8 mg	Available as high potency injectable *(Dilaudid-HP)* and as suppository
Oxymorphone *(Numorphan)*	1.1 mg	3-5	—	Available as suppository
Heroin[4]	4 mg	3-5	—	Adverse effects and dependence liability same as morphine
Agonists related to codeine				
Codeine	130 mg	3-5	30-60 mg	60 mg PO equivalent to 650 mg of aspirin or acetaminophen; usually used orally in combinations with these drugs; dependence liability less than morphine
Dihydrocodeine *(Synalgos-DC; DHCplus)*	—	—	32 mg	Available in combination with aspirin or acetaminophen; dependence liability probably less than morphine
Hydrocodone (*Vicodin*, others)	—	—	5 mg	10 mg PO equivalent to codeine 80 mg PO; available in combination with acetaminophen or aspirin
Oxycodone (*Roxicodone*, others)	—	—	5 mg	10 mg PO equivalent to codeine 90 mg PO; available in combination with acetaminophen or aspirin

Drug	IM dose[1]	IM duration (hours)[2]	Starting oral dose[3]	Comments
Synthetic opioid agonists				
Meperidine (*Demerol*, others)	80 mg	2-4	50 mg	Irritating to tissues IM; toxic metabolite with long half-life causes CNS excitation and convulsions
Fentanyl (*Sublimaze, Duragesic)*	0.1 mg	1-2	—	Used in anesthesia; transdermal patch for chronic pain releases fentanyl over 72 hours
Methadone (*Dolophine*, others)	10 mg	4-6	10-20 mg	Long half-life; risk of CNS depression with repeated use
Propoxyphene HCl (*Darvon*, others)	—	—	65 mg	65 mg of HCl or 100 mg of napsylate PO equivalent to codeine 32 mg PO; available in combinations with acetaminophen or aspirin; toxic metabolite with long half-life causes convulsions and cardiotoxicity; dependence liability less than morphine
Propoxyphene napsylate (*Darvon-N*, others)	—	—	100 mg	
Levorphanol *(Levo-Dromoran)*	1.5-2.5 mg	4-6	2-4 mg	Long half-life; risk of CNS depression with repeated use
Tramadol *(Ultram)*	—	—	50-100 mg	50 mg equivalent to 30 mg of codeine; 100 mg less effective than 650 mg of aspirin plus 60 mg of codeine

(continued)

1. Equivalent to 10 mg of IM morphine
2. With an optimal dose established by titration
3. These drugs are usually given q4-6h, but the duration of action varies with different doses and different patients, and the schedule should be established by titration.
4. Not available for clinical use in USA.

Drug	IM dose[1]	IM duration (hours)[2]	Starting oral dose[3]	Comments
Partial agonists and mixed agonist/antagonists				
Buprenorphine *(Buprenex)*	0.4 mg	4-6	—	Partial agonist; virtually no psychotomimetic effects; sublingual preparation[4] effective
Pentazocine *(Talwin, Talacen)*	60 mg	2-4	50 mg	Mixed agonist/antagonist; 50 mg PO equivalent to codeine 60 mg PO; very irritating to tissues; psychotomimetic effects
Butorphanol *(Stadol, Stadol NS)*	1.5-2.5 mg	3-6	—	Mixed agonist/antagonist; nasal spray produces analgesia comparable to IM injection
Nalbuphine *(Nubain)*	12 mg	3-6	—	Mixed agonist/antagonist; less psychotomimetic effects than pentazocine
Dezocine *(Dalgan)*	10 mg	3-6	—	Mixed agonist/antagonist

1. Equivalent to 10 mg of IM morphine
2. With an optimal dose established by titration
3. These drugs are usually given q4-6h, but the duration of action varies with different doses and different patients, and the schedule should be established by titration.
4. Not available for clinical use in USA.

DRUGS FOR PARKINSON'S DISEASE

New drugs continue to become available for treatment of Parkinson's disease to supplement and ameliorate the effects of levodopa. In the later stages of the disease, there is renewed interest in neurosurgical approaches.

LEVODOPA AND CARBIDOPA — Parkinson's disease is associated with progressive degeneration of dopamine-containing neurons in the substantia nigra. Dopamine itself does not cross the blood-brain barrier and cannot be used to treat Parkinson's disease. Levodopa, the immediate precursor of dopamine, is decarboxylated to dopamine in brain and peripheral tissues. This reaction can be blocked in peripheral tissues by combining levodopa with carbidopa, a peripheral decarboxylase inhibitor. The combination (*Sinemet*, and others) is the most effective treatment available for symptomatic relief of Parkinson's disease.

Limitations – Levodopa is most effective in the first two to five years of treatment. Later, as the disease progresses, the benefit from each dose becomes shorter (the "wearing off" effect), and still later some patients develop sudden, unpredictable fluctuations between mobility and immobility (the "on-off" effect). After about five years of levodopa therapy, many patients have either dose-related clinical fluctuations, dose-related dyskinesias (chorea, dystonia), inadequate response, or toxicity at subtherapeutic dosage. Peripheral adverse effects of levodopa include anorexia, nausea, vomiting, and orthostatic hypotension. Central-nervous-system toxicity including vivid dreams, hallucinations, delusions, confusion and sleep disturbance may occur, especially in older patients. Sudden discontinuation of levodopa for several days may cause not only a return of parkinsonian symptoms, but also a neuroleptic malignant syndrome with fever, rigidity and confusion. Most experts recommend, therefore, tapering the drug over three to four days if possible, rather than stopping it abruptly.

LEVODOPA-CARBIDOPA FORMULATIONS

Carbidopa	Levodopa	Cost*
10 mg	100 mg	
	average generic price (range: $46.80 to $62.30)	$ 53.48
	Sinemet (DuPont Pharma)	62.38
25 mg	100 mg	
	average generic price (range: $51.41 to $62.53)	58.66
	Sinemet (DuPont Pharma)	69.38
	Sinemet CR	70.94
25 mg	250 mg	
	average generic price (range: $54.38 to $83.88)	73.57
	Sinemet (DuPont Pharma)	89.13
50 mg	200 mg	
	Sinemet CR (DuPont Pharma)	146.75

* Cost to the pharmacist for 100 tablets according to wholesale price listings (AWP) in *Drug Topics Red Book* 1995 and May *Update*.

Dosage – The usual daily dosage range is 300 to 1000 mg of levodopa divided into three or four doses; some patients may require up to 2000 mg. Relatively complete inhibition of peripheral decarboxylase requires 75 to 100 mg/day of carbidopa; some patients require doses up to 300 mg to suppress nausea completely. Supplemental carbidopa *(Lodosyn)* is available from the manufacturer of *Sinemet*. Dietary amino acids can decrease the effectiveness of levodopa by competing with the drug for absorption from the intestine and for transport into the brain. The drug may be more effective, therefore, if patients take it at least 30 minutes before eating, and some patients may benefit from a protein-restricted diet. Alternatively, by spreading protein intake evenly throughout the day, patients can take the drug with food, which is helpful in preventing nausea and promotes smoother absorption.

A controlled-release formulation *(Sinemet CR)* is available in two dosages: 50 mg carbidopa with 200 mg of levodopa, and 25 mg carbidopa with 100 mg of levodopa. The higher-dose tablet is scored, but the lower-dose tablet is not, so the smallest possible individual dose is 25/100 mg of carbidopa/levodopa. With its longer half-life, *Sinemet CR* can be beneficial for patients who have wearing-off effects. A disadvantage of *Sinemet CR* is that it takes a longer time to take effect, so many patients take a dose of a standard levodopa-carbidopa combination concurrently, particularly with the first dose in the morning, in order to produce benefit as soon as possible.

Switching to *Sinemet CR* may be difficult for some patients. Because only about 70% of *Sinemet CR* is absorbed, the dosage needs to be about 30% higher than standard levodopa-carbidopa to achieve a comparable effect. Some specialists use *Sinemet CR* instead of the standard formulation when introducing the drug, starting with 25/100 mg once or twice a day, increasing gradually to 25/100 mg t.i.d. or q.i.d. or 50/200 mg b.i.d.

Whether the dosage and duration of levodopa use contribute to the long-term complications of the disease is unclear. Most experts advise using levodopa only when symptoms become functionally limiting without it.

SELEGILINE ***(Eldepryl)*** — Another drug widely used for treatment of Parkinson's disease is selegiline, an irreversible inhibitor of monoamine oxidase type B (MAO-B) also known as deprenyl (Medical Letter, 31:81, 1989). Treatment with selegiline in early Parkinson's disease before levodopa is introduced can delay the need for levodopa for six to nine months, probably because of a mild beneficial effect on parkinsonian symptoms (Parkinson Study Group, N Engl J Med, 328:176, 1993). There is no convincing evidence that selegiline slows the progression of Parkinson's disease. Some clinicians begin treatment with selegiline as soon as the diagnosis has been made, reserving levodopa until symptoms become disabling. The usual dosage is 5 mg with breakfast and at lunch; to decrease the risk of insomnia (selegiline is metabolized to methamphetamine and amphetamine), the drug should not be taken later in the day.

The cost of one month's treatment with *Eldepryl*, 5 mg b.i.d., is $128.19, according to *Drugs Topics Red Book* May 1995 *Update*. Nausea and orthostatic hypotension may occur. Selegiline in recommended doses, unlike MAO-A inhibitors used for treatment of depression, does not cause hypertension after ingestion of tyramine-rich foods or with concomitant levodopa therapy. The drug has, however, caused toxic interactions with tricyclic antidepressants such as amitryptiline (*Elavil*, and others), selective serotonin reuptake inhibitors (SSRIs) such as fluoxetine *(Prozac)* and with meperidine (*Demerol*, and others) (O Suchowersky and JD deVries, Can J Psychiatry, 35:571, 1990; GL Zornberg et al, Lancet, 337:246, 1991; JL Montastruc et al, Lancet, 341:555, 1993; FDA Med Bull, 25:6, 1995).

Because selegiline inhibits catabolism of dopamine in the brain, it can potentiate the effect of levodopa and increase levodopa toxicity, particularly psychosis and dyskinesia.

DOPAMINE AGONISTS — Two ergot-derivative dopamine agonists, bromocriptine *(Parlodel)* and pergolide (*Permax* – Medical Letter, 31:81, 1989), are currently marketed in the USA mainly for adjunctive (with levodopa) treatment of Parkinson's disease; lisuride is available in some other countries. These drugs have less antiparkinson effect than levodopa used alone, but they are less likely to cause dyskinesias and have a longer duration of action (MA Hely et al, J Neurol Neurosurg Psychiatry, 57:903, 1994). Used as an adjunct to levodopa, dopamine agonists may contribute to clinical improvement while permitting a reduction in levodopa dosage (CW Olanow et al, Mov Disord, 9:40, 1994). Used alone, they may permit a delay in introduction of levodopa and in the occurrence of complications associated with long-term levodopa use (JL Montastruc, J Neurol Neurosurg Psychiatry, 57:1034, 1994).

Dopamine agonists can cause nausea and postural hypotension, which may limit their use. Some Medical Letter consultants recommend starting with 1.25 mg of bromocriptine daily for the first three days, then increasing slowly to 15 to 30 mg per day, divided b.i.d. or t.i.d. with meals. The recommended dosage of pergolide is 0.05 mg per day for the first three days, then increasing slowly to 1.5 to 3 mg per day, divided t.i.d. Dopamine agonists, like selegiline, can potentiate dyskinesias or toxic psychosis caused by levodopa. As the dosage of the dopamine agonist increases, levodopa dosage may have to be decreased to avoid such effects. Even when used alone, the dopamine agonists can cause confusion and toxic psychosis.

Peripheral dopaminergic effects, such as nausea, can be blocked by the dopamine antagonist domperidone *(Motilium)*, which is available in Canada but not the USA. Ergot-related adverse effects such as erythromelalgia, edema, pain, and digital spasms in the extremities have occurred with dopamine agonists. Pleural effusions, fibrotic pulmonary changes and retroperitoneal fibrosis have been reported rarely.

Apomorphine, a potent dopamine agonist available in Canada, injected subcutaneously can rapidly reverse the sudden "off" state seen in some patients with advanced Parkinson's disease after long-term levodopa therapy (AJ Hughes et al, Mov Disord, 8:165, 1993). Apomorphine causes emesis, but oral domperidone started 48 hours before treatment blocks the emetic effect. A long-acting dopamine agonist (cabergoline) is an investigational drug in the USA (A Lieberman et al, Neurology, 43:1981, 1993).

CATECHOL-O-METHYLTRANSFERASE INHIBITORS — Levodopa is metabolized by two enzymes, dopa decarboxylase and catechol-O-methyltransferase (COMT). Two inhibitors of COMT, tolcapone and entacapone, are currently undergoing clinical trials. Used in combination with levodopa, these drugs have been reported to increase the plasma half-life of levodopa and to decrease parkinsonian disability and the amount of "off" time, but they also increase dyskinesias (JW Roberts et al, Neurology, 43:2685, 1994; S Kaakkola et al, Neurology, 44:77, 1994; M Merello et al, J Neurol Neurosurg Psychiatry, 57:186, 1994).

ANTICHOLINERGICS — In Parkinson's disease, the decreased activity of dopamine makes the excitatory effects of acetylcholine more prominent. Before levodopa, anticholinergic agents were the only drugs available to treat Parkinson's disease, and they are still useful in some patients, especially for treatment of tremor and drooling. Although not as effective as levodopa or dopamine agonists, they may have an additive therapeutic effect at any stage of the disease. Adverse effects of anticholinergic drugs include dry mouth, constipation, urinary retention, aggravation of glaucoma, impaired memory, confusion and hallucinations; these may be more prominent in elderly patients. Anticholinergics available in the USA include trihexyphenidyl (*Artane*; and others), benztropine (*Cogentin*, and others), procyclidine *(Kemadrin)*, and biperiden *(Akineton)*. Antihistamines such as diphenhydramine (*Benadryl*, and others) also have anticholinergic effects and are occasionally useful for patients who cannot tolerate the more potent anticholinergics. Abrupt discontinuation of any of these drugs can cause severe exacerbation of symptoms.

AMANTADINE — Amantadine (*Symmetrel*, and others), mainly an antiviral drug, in parkinsonism may increase release of dopamine in the brain. In a dosage of 100 mg b.i.d. or t.i.d., it has been used alone to treat early Parkinson's disease, or as an adjunct in later stages. Some patients may not respond to amantadine, but the drug should be taken for about two weeks before assuming it is ineffective. Confusion and hallucinations, ankle edema, and livedo reticularis can occur. Amantadine is not metabolized, but is excreted in urine; dosage must be decreased for patients with renal dysfunction. High serum concentrations of amantadine cause a severe psychosis. Amantadine and anticholinergics may have additive adverse effects on mental function. Sudden withdrawal of amantadine can cause severe exacerbation of parkinsonian symptoms or neuroleptic malignant syndrome (DJ Bower et al, Am J Psychiatry, 151:451, 1994).

ANTIDEPRESSANTS — Depression commonly accompanies Parkinson's disease and must be treated, if present, for the patient to benefit adequately from antiparkinson drugs. The drug of choice is usually a tricyclic antidepressant or trazodone *(Desyrel)*. Experience with fluoxetine *(Prozac)* or other selective serotonin reuptake inhibitors is more limited; worsening of Parkinson's symptoms has been reported (ENH Jansen Steur, Neurology, 43:211, 1993; FJ Jimenez-Jimenez et al, Neurology, 44:2406, 1994). MAO-A inhibitors should not be used because they can cause marked swings in blood pressure in patients taking levodopa.

CLOZAPINE — Clozapine is an antipsychotic drug that only rarely causes drug-induced parkinsonism, making it particularly useful in controlling psychosis associated with levodopa or dopamine agonists in patients with Parkinson's disease (JM Rabey et al, Neurology, 45:432, 1995). Doses of clozapine lower than those usually needed to treat schizophrenia are effective in levodopa-induced psychosis. Drowsiness is a common adverse effect. The dosage is 6.25 or 12.5 mg h.s., which can be increased gradually until psychosis is controlled. The drug has also been used to suppress tremor and dyskinesias in patients with Parkinson's disease (ENH Jansen, Acta Neurol Scand, 89:262, 1994; JP Bennett, Jr et al, Mov Disord, 9:409, 1994). Because clozapine can cause agranulocytosis in 1% to 2% of patients, weekly blood counts are necessary.

CISAPRIDE — Cisapride (*Propulsid* – Medical Letter, 36:11, 1994), a prokinetic drug marketed for treatment of gastroesophageal reflux has been used to treat constipation in patients with Parkinson's disease (WH Jost and K Schimrigk, Mov Disord, 8:339, 1993). By accelerating gastric emptying, cisapride can also shorten the time it takes for levodopa to become effective from an average of 60 minutes to 45 minutes after the first morning dose (R Djaldetti et al, Mov Disord, 10:81, 1995).

VITAMIN E — A multicenter controlled trial found that vitamin E (tocopherol), used in the hope that its antioxidant effect would delay progression of Parkinson's disease, was not effective (Parkinson Study Group, N Engl J Med, 328:176, 1993).

SURGICAL TREATMENT — Several surgical techniques have been tried for treatment of Parkinson's disease (Medical Letter, 35:103, 1993). Transplantation of dopaminergic cells from human fetal brain tissue may decrease the severity of the disease and permit use of lower doses of levodopa (O Lindvall et al, Ann Neurol, 35:172, 1994; JH Kordower et al, N Engl J Med, 332:1118, 1995).

Unilateral ablation of the ventral intermediate nucleus of the thalamus can abolish contralateral tremor in 80% of patients, with serious neurological complications in less than 10%. In some of these patients, improvement has been sustained for more than 10 years. However, if tremor is severe bilaterally, requiring bilateral lesions, complications occur more frequently (RR Tasker, Neurosurg Clin North Am, 1:841, 1990).

Pallidotomy, ablation of the posteroventral portion of the globus pallidus, appears to be effective in controlling dyskinesias, and unilateral pallidotomy, for reasons not yet understood, appears to control dyskinesia bilaterally to some extent. Pallidotomy also has some effect in controlling bradykinesia, rigidity, tremor and ambulatory difficulties (RP Iacono et al, Am Surg, 60:777, 1994).

High frequency electrical stimulation through implanted electrodes in the ventral intermediate nucleus of the thalamus has been reported to control contralateral tremor and levodopa-induced dyskinesias (D Caparros-Lefebvre et al, J Neurol Neurosurg Psychiatry, 56:268, 1993). Stimulation of the subthalamic nucleus bilaterally has been reported to improve motor function (P Limousin et al, Lancet, 345:91, 1995).

CONCLUSION — Levodopa combined with carbidopa is the most effective symptomatic treatment for Parkinson's disease, but many clinicians withhold it early in the disease in an attempt to ameliorate the limitations and complications of long-term use. Some neurologists prescribe selegiline as soon as the diagnosis of Parkinson's disease has been established to delay the need for levodopa, and concurrent use of the two drugs may permit use of lower levodopa dosage. Dopamine agonists, which are the next most powerful drugs after levodopa in decreasing the symptoms of Parkinson's disease, can be used alone in an attempt to delay the introduction of levodopa or as an adjunct to levodopa.

DRUGS FOR PSYCHIATRIC DISORDERS

Many drugs are available for treatment of psychiatric disorders, and it is often difficult to choose among them. The recommendations in this article are based on the results of controlled trials and on the experience and opinions of Medical Letter consultants. Adverse effects of these drugs are listed in the table beginning on page 145. Interactions with other drugs can be found in *The Medical Letter Handbook of Adverse Drug Interactions*, 1995.

DRUGS FOR ANXIETY — When anxiety is a symptom of another psychiatric syndrome, such as depression or psychosis, the specific treatment for the syndrome is generally more effective than use of nonspecific anxiolytic agents, such as benzodiazepines. Anxiety that requires drug treatment and is not related to a more specific syndrome is usually treated with a benzodiazepine. Diazepam (*Valium*, and others), chlordiazepoxide (*Librium*, and others), alprazolam *(Xanax)*, clorazepate (*Tranxene*, and others), halazepam *(Paxipam)*, lorazepam (*Ativan*, and others), oxazepam (*Serax*, and others) and prazepam are similar in their clinical effects, although they differ in pharmacokinetics (RI Shader and DJ Greenblatt, N Engl J Med, 328:1398, 1993). Clonazepam *(Klonopin)*, a long-acting benzodiazepine approved by the US Food and Drug Administration (FDA) only for treatment of epilepsy, is also sometimes used for treatment of anxiety and other psychiatric symptoms. For treatment of chronic anxiety, buspirone *(BuSpar)*, a non-benzodiazepine anti-anxiety drug (Medical Letter, 28:117, 1986), does not cause sedation and has no known potential for abuse; it may, however, take as long as four weeks to act, and some Medical Letter consultants question its effectiveness.

For prevention of panic attacks, alprazolam is the only drug approved by the FDA, but most Medical Letter consultants now use low doses of a selective serotonin reuptake inhibitor (SSRI) such as fluoxetine *(Prozac)*; usual doses of an SSRI can exacerbate panic attacks (AK Louie et al, J Clin Psychiatry, 54:435, 1993). Propranolol (*Inderal*, and others) and other beta-blockers have been used to prevent the symptoms of performance anxiety or "stage fright" (R Pohl et al, J Clin Psychopharmacol, 8:225, 1988). Another anxiety disorder that may respond to drug treatment is social phobia (*Diagnostic and Statistical Manual of Mental Disorders*, 4th ed [DSM-IV], Washington, DC:American Psychiatric Association, 1994, page 411); monoamine oxidase (MAO) inhibitors, benzodiazepines and SSRIs have been tried with some success (RD Marshall et al, J Clin Psychiatry, 55, no. 6 suppl:33, 1994).

Adverse Effects – Sedation is the most common adverse effect of the benzodiazepines; it may be more severe in the elderly and increase the risk of falls. Anterograde amnesia, inability to remember a period of hours after taking the drug, has occurred in some patients. Oral overdoses of benzodiazepines taken alone are rarely lethal, but they can be dangerous if taken with alcohol, barbiturates, opioids or other drugs that depress the central nervous system (CNS). In patients with compromised respiration, any CNS depressant, including a benzodiazepine, may be dangerous. Flumazenil *(Mazicon)* is an effective antidote for benzodiazepine oversedation (Medical Letter, 34:66, 1992).

Withdrawal – Physical dependence may develop with chronic use of benzodiazepines. Recurrent anxiety and withdrawal symptoms (insomnia, nausea, vomiting, twitching, sweating, delirium, muscle cramps, irritability, tinnitus, paresthesias and, rarely, convulsions) have developed when these drugs were abruptly discontinued, especially after prolonged or excessive use. Symptoms may be especially common after discontinuation of alprazolam or lorazepam. Gradual tapering of dosage, sometimes over weeks or months, is recommended. With some benzodiazepines that have long half-lives, such as chlordiazepoxide, diazepam or clorazepate, withdrawal symptoms and rebound anxiety may be less frequent and milder.

DRUGS FOR DEPRESSION — Major depressive disorders often require treatment with drugs, but the diagnosis is sometimes obscured by anxiety, insomnia, substance abuse or the multiple somatic complaints that frequently accompany depression. Many drugs can also cause depression (Medical Letter, 35:65, 1993).

Severe depression in the elderly may be associated with prominent cognitive symptoms ("pseudodementia") and may sometimes be confused with an organic mental syndrome. Severely depressed patients with delusions or other psychotic symptoms require an antipsychotic drug concurrently with an antidepressant. Electroconvulsive therapy (ECT) can be highly effective for treatment of depression, especially for psychotic and elderly patients.

Choice of Drugs – In the past, a tricyclic antidepressant such as imipramine (*Tofranil*, and others), amitryptiline (*Elavil*, and others), or nortriptyline (*Pamelor*, and others) has generally been considered the drug of first choice for treatment of nonpsychotic, nonbipolar depression. Now, however, an SSRI such as fluoxetine *(Prozac)*, sertraline *(Zoloft)*, or paroxetine *(Paxil)* is often used instead, particularly for patients with mild to moderate depression (Medical Letter, 35:25, 1993). MAO inhibitors, such as phenelzine *(Nardil)* or tranylcypromine *(Parnate)*, are effective antidepressants that can be helpful for some patients who cannot tolerate or fail to respond to a tricyclic antidepressant or SSRI. Bupropion (*Wellbutrin* – Medical Letter, 31:97, 1989) and venlafaxine (*Effexor* – Medical Letter 36:49, 1994) are additional alternatives that may be effective for some patients. All of these drugs require several weeks for maximum therapeutic benefit.

Trazodone *(Desyrel)* can be helpful as a second drug for patients with SSRI-associated sleep disturbances (AA Nierenberg, Am J Psychiatry, 151:1069, 1994). Adding lithium, triiodothyronine, a stimulant or a second antidepressant of a different class to adequate doses of a tricyclic or other antidepressant may be effective in some patients with refractory unipolar depression (JC Nelson, J Clin Psychiatry, 54, no. 9 suppl:42, 1993; RT Joffe et al, Arch Gen Psychiatry, 50:387, 1993). Nefazodone *(Serzone)* is a new antidepressant (Medical Letter, 37:33, 1995) that inhibits reuptake of serotonin and norepinephrine; available data are inadequate to determine how it compares with other antidepressants.

Adverse Effects – The most common adverse reactions that limit treatment with tricyclic antidepressants are anticholinergic effects, orthostatic hypotension, sedation, sexual dysfunction and weight gain. In children, adolescents, and young adults, tricyclics may cause tachycardia and mild hypertension (BT Walsh et al, J Clin Psychopharmacol, 12:163, 1992). Elderly patients are more sensitive to the anticholinergic effects of tricyclics and may develop delirium with high doses or when they are taking other anticholinergic drugs concurrently. Tricyclics also have quinidine-like effects on the heart; another type of antidepressant may be preferable for patients with pre-existing delayed ventricular conduction or other cardiac problems (AH Glassman et al, JAMA, 269:2673, 1993). Overdosage with a tricyclic can be lethal; serious reactions are characterized by heart block, cardiac arrhythmias, hypotension, convulsions and coma. Amitriptyline tends to cause a high incidence of sedative and anticholinergic effects. Desipramine therapy has been associated with rare instances of sudden cardiac death in children (MA Riddle et al, J Am Acad Child Adolesc Psychiatry, 32:792, 1993). Amoxapine (*Asendin*, and others) has been associated with development of extrapyramidal effects, tardive dyskinesia, and the neuroleptic malignant syndrome. Withdrawal symptoms (gastrointestinal upset, dizziness, headache, malaise, increased perspiration, nightmares, and salivation) have been reported after abruptly stopping treatment with a tricyclic; dosage should be tapered when these drugs are stopped after long-term use.

SSRIs such as fluoxetine, paroxetine, and sertraline cause nausea, headache, nervousness and insomnia more commonly than the tricyclics, but generally do not cause weight gain, are less likely to cause anticholinergic effects or orthostatic hypotension, and are much safer in overdosage. Agitation and increased anxiety may occur in the first weeks of treatment. All SSRIs appear to cause a high incidence of anorgasmia and other sexual dysfunction. Akathisia can be troublesome and may be more common with fluoxetine. Concurrent use of fluoxetine with tricyclics or other drugs metabolized by the cytochrome P450 hepatic enzyme system can lead to increased concentrations of the other drugs, sometimes to toxic levels (*Medical Letter Handbook of Adverse Drug Interactions*, 1995, p 253); interactions may also occur with paroxetine, but seem to be less of a problem with sertraline.

Bupropion may cause agitation and, rarely, seizures, but causes fewer anticholinergic effects than the tricyclic antidepressants, little if any orthostatic hypotension, and a relatively low incidence of sexual dysfunction. Venlafaxine generally is similar to the SSRIs in its adverse effects, but it has been associated with a sustained increase in diastolic blood pressure. Trazodone is sedating and can cause priapism in men, sometimes leading to permanent loss of erectile function. Maprotiline (*Ludiomil*, and others) has been associated with an increased risk of seizures. Nefazodone can cause headache, somnolence and postural hypotension.

Patients taking MAO inhibitors should be warned that they interact with many other drugs and can cause a hypertensive crisis when taken concurrently with levodopa (*Larodopa*, and others), sympathomimetic amines found in many over-the-counter preparations marketed for treatment of colds, weight loss, etc., or with tyramine-rich foods or beverages (see table on page 150). Concurrent use of an MAO inhibitor with buspirone can also cause hypertension. Spontaneous acute hypertensive reactions have even occurred in patients taking an MAO inhibitor alone, possibly due to conversion of the drug to metabolites with pressor activity. When a pounding occipital headache develops, taking 10 mg of nifedipine (*Procardia*, and others) can lower blood pressure and relieve the symptoms (DH Golwyn and CP Sevlie, J Clin Psychopharmacol, 13:77, 1993).

Use of a tricyclic antidepressant, an SSRI, meperidine (*Demerol*, and others) or the cough suppressant dextromethorphan in a patient already taking an MAO inhibitor may lead to delirium, hyperpyrexia, convulsions, coma and death. When transferring a patient from a tricyclic to an MAO inhibitor, a drug-free interval of one week is recommended. When changing from fluoxetine to an MAO inhibitor, the recommended drug-free interval is five weeks or possibly longer (MT Pato et al, J Clin Psychopharmacol, 11:224, 1991); two weeks is sufficient when changing from sertraline or paroxetine. When changing from an MAO inhibitor to a tricyclic or SSRI, a two-week interval is recommended. Abrupt withdrawal of an MAO inhibitor can cause psychosis, delirium, tachycardia, insomnia and nightmares. Overdosage with an MAO inhibitor can cause hypotension, convulsions and death.

OBSESSIVE-COMPULSIVE DISORDER — Clomipramine (*Anafranil,* fluoxetine and fluvoxamine (*Luvox* – Medical Letter, 37:13, 1995) have been approved by the FDA for treatment of obsessive-compulsive disorder (DSM-IV, page 417). Other tricyclics and SSRIs may also be helpful for this condition (MA Jenike, Psychiatr Clin North Am, 15:895, 1992).

DRUGS FOR MANIA — Lithium (*Eskalith,* and others) is the standard treatment for mania and bipolar depression and the drug of choice for long-term maintenance to prevent both manic and depressive episodes in patients with bipolar disorder (LH Price and GR Heninger, N Engl J Med, 331:591, 1994). Lithium may take two to four weeks to have a full therapeutic effect; acutely manic patients often require temporary treatment with an antipsychotic drug such as haloperidol or a benzodiazepine such as lorazepam. During depressive episodes, an antidepressant is often needed temporarily in addition to lithium, but may precipitate mania. Lithium can be given safely if serum concentrations are monitored; they should be measured about 12 hours after the last dose. For long-term maintenance, serum concentrations between 0.8 and 1.0 mEq/L provide more protection against recurrent mood episodes than lower concentrations (0.4 to 0.6 mEq/L), but with a higher incidence of adverse effects. For many patients, serum concentrations of 0.6 or 0.7 mEq/L are effective and well tolerated.

Adverse Effects – Nausea and fatigue may occur in the first weeks of treatment with lithium, even when serum concentrations are in the recommended range. Tremor, thirst, polyuria, edema, and weight gain may persist for the duration of treatment. Lithium-induced tremors can be treated by lowering dosage or adding a beta-blocker. Confusion and ataxia are important toxic effects of lithium that may not be perceived as drug-induced. Toxic renal effects, including tubular lesions, interstitial fibrosis and decreased creatinine clearance have been reported in patients treated chronically with lithium, but are uncommon. Nephrogenic diabetes insipidus is a renal complication that can persist for months or years in some patients. Thyroid disturbances, primarily mild hypothyroidism, are fairly common. Lithium may cause mild leukocytosis, can induce or exacerbate psoriasis, and can cause severe acne, folliculitis and other skin reactions.

Lithium should be given with caution to elderly patients, those with dementia, patients with cardiac disease, decreased sodium intake or increased sodium losses, and to those taking nonsteroidal anti-inflammatory drugs. Lithium taken during pregnancy may cause a cardiac malformation in the fetus (LS Cohen et al, JAMA, 271:146, 1994).

Alternatives – For patients who cannot tolerate lithium, the anticonvulsant valproic acid (*Depakene, Depakote,* and others) may be the best alternative for treatment of mania (Medical Letter, 36:74, 1994). One controlled trial in patients with acute mania found valproate as effective as lithium and much more effective than placebo (CL Bowden et al, JAMA, 271:918, 1994). An ongoing multicenter study is assessing the effectiveness of valproate in long-term prevention of recurrent episodes of mania. The anticonvulsants carbamazepine (*Tegretol,* and others) and clonazepam *(Klonopin)* have also been used to treat patients with bipolar disorder (C Van Valkenburg et al, Drugs, 44:326, 1992). ECT is effective for treatment of both acute mania and acute depression. An antipsychotic drug alone can be given to treat manic episodes and an antidepressant to treat depression, but an antidepressant, especially without lithium, may precipitate mania in patients with bipolar disorder.

PSYCHOSES — Some symptoms of schizophrenia and acute psychoses may improve rapidly after treatment with antipsychotic drugs, but chronic schizophrenia usually improves slowly over many weeks and may continue to improve for months. Many patients with chronic schizophrenia require prolonged maintenance therapy, but the risk of tardive movement disorders must be kept in mind. Acute psychotic episodes associated with endocrinologic or metabolic disturbance, drug reactions (particularly to corticosteroids), or psychiatric conditions other than schizophrenia can usually be managed symptomatically with an antipsychotic drug, if specific therapy for the underlying disorder is not effective.

Drugs – Haloperidol and the phenothiazines listed in the table on pages 146 to 148 are all about equally effective in previously untreated patients, but clozapine *(Clozaril)* may relieve symptoms in some schizophrenic patients resistant to treatment with other antipsychotics and may produce a better quality of response (Medical Letter, 35:16, 1993). Risperidone *(Risperdal)*, the newest antipsychotic drug, also appears to be effective for treatment of chronic schizophrenia with a low rate of extrapyramidal effects (Medical Letter, 36:33, 1994).

For emergency treatment of agitated schizophrenic patients, concurrent use of a benzodiazepine and haloperidol may be effective (JG Barbee et al, Am J Psychiatry, 149:506, 1992). When a long-acting parenteral antipsychotic drug is indicated, usually to improve compliance with maintenance therapy, fluphenazine decanoate (*Prolixin*, and others) or haloperidol decanoate *(Haldol Decanoate)* can be used (WM Glazer and JM Kane, J Clin Psychiatry, 53:426, 1992).

Adverse Effects – Chlorpromazine causes sedation, postural hypotension, weight gain, and anticholinergic and occasional extrapyramidal effects. Thioridazine (*Mellaril*, and others) causes fewer acute extrapyramidal reactions than most other antipsychotics, but it is sedating, has marked anticholinergic activity, and can cause hypotension, delayed cardiac conduction time, a prolonged QT-interval (and possibly the torsades de pointes ventricular arrhythmia), disturbances of ejaculation and, in doses higher than 600 to 800 mg daily, can cause pigmentary retinopathy. Weight gain is less common with molindone *(Moban)* than with other antipsychotic drugs. Hypotension and sedation are less likely with perphenazine (*Trilafon*, and others), fluphenazine (*Prolixin*, and others), trifluoperazine (*Stelazine*, and others), thiothixene (*Navane*, and others) or haloperidol, but all of these drugs tend to cause frequent extrapyramidal reactions.

Parkinson-like extrapyramidal effects of antipsychotic drugs that cannot be relieved by lowering the dosage can be treated with anticholinergic antiparkinson drugs such as benztropine mesylate (*Cogentin*, and others) or trihexyphenidyl (*Artane*, and others). Amantadine (*Symmetrel*, and others), an antiparkinson drug that is not primarily anticholinergic, can also be useful for this purpose, but can accumulate and cause toxic effects in patients with decreased renal function. Acute dystonic reactions, such as oculogyric crisis or torticollis, can be treated with a single injection of

50 mg of diphenhydramine (*Benadryl*, and others), followed by days to weeks of oral treatment. Akathisia (intense restlessness) is a common extrapyramidal reaction that may not respond to anticholinergics but may respond to propranolol (LA Adler et al, Psychopharmacol Bull, 29:283, 1993).

Tardive movement disorders, characterized by involuntary movements and sustained postures, initially of the face, eyes, lips, and tongue, but sometimes also of the fingers, toes or trunk, are serious late effects of drugs used to treat schizophrenia; they usually occur after prolonged therapy and sometimes persist for long periods or for life, even after the drug is discontinued. Rarely, they occur less than a year after beginning treatment. Because of the possibility of these reactions, the lowest effective dosage of antipsychotic drugs should be used. Many drugs have been tried for treatment of tardive dyskinesia or dystonia; none has been established as effective, but clozapine might prove to be beneficial (JA Lieberman et al, Br J Psychiatry, 158: 503, 1991).

The neuroleptic malignant syndrome, characterized by hyperthermia, akinesia, muscle rigidity, autonomic instability and altered consciousness, is an uncommon but potentially lethal reaction to antipsychotic drugs. It can occur early in the course of treatment, especially with high doses.

Clozapine apparently does not cause acute extrapyramidal reactions or tardive movement disorders, and may improve the abnormal movements of tardive dyskinesia and tardive dystonia. The drug does, however, cause granulocytopenia or agranulocytosis in about 1% to 2% of patients; with weekly monitoring of blood counts, fatalities are rare (JMJ Alvir et al, N Engl J Med, 329:162, 1993). Granulocyte colony-stimulating factor may be useful in treating agranulocytosis due to clozapine (CB Geibig and LW Marks, Ann Pharmacother, 27:1190, 1993; H Nielsen, J Intern Med, 234:529, 1993).

Risperidone is a new drug, and determination of its adverse effects may still be incomplete. It can cause asthenia, sedation, and difficulty in concentrating. Orthostatic hypotension and reflex tachycardia can occur initially, especially in the elderly. Elevation of serum prolactin levels, weight gain and sexual dysfunction have been reported. The incidence of extrapyramidal effects is dose-dependent, but in patients taking recommended doses of risperidone has been only slightly higher than with placebo. Neither tardive dyskinesia nor agranulocytosis has been reported in patients taking risperidone. Interactions with other drugs also have not been reported.

"ORGANIC" MENTAL DISORDER — Syndromes with features of stupor, delirium or dementia occur most often in older patients with Alzheimer's disease or other degenerative disorders. In younger patients, they may be due to alcohol or drug abuse or withdrawal, a reaction to a drug or its withdrawal, electrolyte or other metabolic imbalance, or to a cerebral tumor, injury or infection. Hospitalized, older patients without recognized dementia often become confused, disoriented and agitated.

Drugs – Some clinicians prescribe a benzodiazepine for agitated patients, particularly if they suspect a withdrawal reaction, but these drugs sometimes add to the patient's confusion. Unlike schizophrenia, organic mental syndromes often respond within hours to low doses of a relatively nonsedating antipsychotic (such as perphenazine, fluphenazine or haloperidol), but larger doses of antipsychotics may be too sedating or cause movement disorders. Some consultants recommend a phenothiazine such as thioridazine, which is sedating but usually causes few extrapyramidal symptoms; thioridazine may, however, cause moderate to severe postural hypotension and has significant anticholinergic effects, which may make confusion worse. Haloperidol, which has few autonomic effects but frequent extrapyramidal effects, may be safer for patients with cardiovascular problems. Many clinicians use both an antipsychotic and a benzodiazepine when either alone has been ineffective.

ADVERSE EFFECTS OF PSYCHIATRIC DRUGS

ALPRAZOLAM *(Xanax)*
see Benzodiazepines

AMITRIPTYLINE (*Elavil*, and others)
see Tricyclic antidepressants

AMOXAPINE (*Asendin*, and others)
see Tricyclic antidepressants

BENZODIAZEPINES (alprazolam, chlordiazepoxide, clonazepam, clorazepate, diazepam, halazepam, lorazepam, oxazepam, prazepam, temazepam)
Frequent: Drowsiness; ataxia
Occasional: Confusion; amnesia; disinhibition; paradoxical excitement; depression; dizziness; withdrawal symptoms, including delirium and convulsions, on abrupt discontinuance (withdrawal may be especially difficult with alprazolam); rebound insomnia or excitement
Rare: Hypotension; blood dyscrasias; jaundice; allergic reactions; paradoxical rage reactions; stuttering with alprazolam

BUPROPION *(Wellbutrin)*
Frequent: Anxiety; agitation; insomnia; tremor, anorexia
Occasional: Seizures (dose-related)
Rare: Mania; falling backward; tinnitus; hallucinations

BUSPIRONE *(BuSpar)*
Frequent: Dizziness; headache
Occasional: Nausea; paresthesias; diarrhea
Rare: Psychosis; mania

CARBAMAZEPINE (*Tegretol*, and others)
Frequent: Drowsiness; dizziness; ataxia; nausea; vomiting; rash
Occasional: Confusion; blurred vision; diplopia; headache; leukopenia; thrombocytopenia
Rare: Agranulocytosis; aplastic anemia; Stevens-Johnson syndrome; cardiac toxicity; antidiuretic effect; aseptic meningitis; hepatitis

CHLORDIAZEPOXIDE (*Librium*, and others) see Benzodiazepines

CHLORPROMAZINE (*Thorazine*, and others) see Phenothiazines, aliphatic

CHLORPROTHIXENE *(Taractan)*
similar to Phenothiazines, aliphatic

CLOMIPRAMINE *(Anafranil)*
see Tricyclic antidepressants

CLONAZEPAM *(Klonopin)*
see Benzodiazepines

CLORAZEPATE (*Tranxene*, and others), see Benzodiazepines

CLOZAPINE *(Clozaril)*
Frequent: Drowsiness; constipation; anticholinergic effects;* postural hypotension; increase in body temperature; increased salivation; EKG changes; weight gain
Occasional: Hypertension; granulocytopenia; agranulocytosis; seizures
Rare: Hyponatremia; pancreatitis; cardiorespiratory collapse; neuroleptic malignant syndrome

---

* Dry mouth, mydriasis, cycloplegia, urinary retention, decreased GI motility, tachycardia, memory impairment and, in high doses, delirium

DESIPRAMINE (*Norpramin*, and others) see Tricyclic antidepressants

DIAZEPAM (*Valium*, and others), see Benzodiazepines

DOXEPIN (*Adapin*, and others), see Tricyclic antidepressants

FLUOXETINE *(Prozac)*

Frequent: Nausea; nervousness; headache; insomnia; sexual dysfunction (anorgasmia)

Occasional: Akathisia; rash; fever; arthralgia; mania; aminotransferase elevations; abulia; alopecia

Rare: Extrapyramidal reactions; seizures in patients with preexisting seizure disorder; leukocytosis; bradycardia with syncope; respiratory distress; anorexia; serum sickness; platelet dysfunction and bleeding; penile anesthesia; psoriasis; cognitive dysfunction; antidiuresis

FLUPHENAZINE (*Permitil, Prolixin*, and others) see Phenothiazines, piperazine

HALAZEPAM *(Paxipam)*, see Benzodiazepines

HALOPERIDOL (*Haldol*, and others)

Frequent: Extrapyramidal effects (especially in young patients)

Occasional: Blood dyscrasias; postural hypotension; sedation; menstrual changes; galactorrhea; tardive dyskinesia

Rare: Cholestatic jaundice; photosensitivity; rash; weight gain; convulsions; impotence; neurotoxicity in hyperthyroid patients; neuroleptic malignant syndrome

IMIPRAMINE (*Tofranil*, and others) see Tricyclic antidepressants

LITHIUM (*Eskalith*, and others)

At therapeutic serum concentrations (0.6 – 1.2 mEq/L): Thirst; polyuria; fine tremor; GI irritation; mild diarrhea; weight gain; edema; leukocytosis

At toxic serum concentrations (above 2 mEq/L): Confusion; vomiting; diarrhea; polyuria; muscle weakness; ataxia; lethargy; slurred speech; tinnitus; blurred vision; nystagmus; stupor; coma; convulsions; permanent neurologic impairment

Occasional (at all serum concentrations): Goiter; hypothyroidism; nephrogenic diabetes insipidus; acne; renal tubular acidosis; metallic taste; induction or exacerbation of psoriasis; folliculitis; T-wave changes; nausea; extrapyramidal effects

Rare (at all serum concentrations): Exophthalmos; cardiac arrhythmias; vomiting; acute renal failure; progressive decrease in renal function; Raynaud's phenomenon; hypoglycemia; hair loss; pseudotumor cerebri; hyperthyroidism; hyperparathyroidism; thrombocytopenia; keratodermia; erythema multiforme

(Note: Serum concentrations and toxic effects increased by dehydration, diuretics, sweating, fever, protracted diarrhea or diminished intake of sodium)

LORAZEPAM (*Ativan*, and others), see Benzodiazepines

LOXAPINE (*Loxitane*, and others) similar to Phenothiazines, piperazine

MAO INHIBITORS (phenelzine, tranylcypromine)

Frequent: Hypotension; restlessness; insomnia; daytime sleepiness

Occasional: Mania; urinary retention; tremors; sexual disturbances; paresthesias; dry mouth; nausea; constipation; anorexia; weight gain; edema; withdrawal symptoms

Rare: Rash; hepatitis; tinnitus; muscle spasm; lupus-like reaction; leukopenia; hyperthermia; hypertension

(Note: Interactions with drugs or foods may be severe)

MAPROTILINE (*Ludiomil*, others)

Similar to tricyclics, but seizures occur more frequently (especially with more than 200 mg/day) and anticholinergic effects* may occur less frequently

MESORIDAZINE *(Serentil)*, see Phenothiazines, piperidine

MOLINDONE *(Moban)*

Frequent: Extrapyramidal effects; akathisia; anticholinergic effects*

Occasional: Drowsiness; dystonia; menstrual changes; anorexia; weight loss; rash; tardive dyskinesia

Rare: Leukopenia; postural hypotension; ECG abnormalities; liver abnormalities; neuroleptic malignant syndrome

NEFAZODONE *(Serzone)*

Occasional: Headache; somnolence; dry mouth; nausea; dizziness; blurred vision; impotence; anorgasmia

NORTRIPTYLINE *(Aventyl*, and others) see Tricyclic antidepressants

OXAZEPAM (*Serax*, and others), see Benzodiazepines

PAROXETINE *(Paxil)*

Frequent: Nausea; sweating; asthenia; somnolence; dizziness; insomnia; tremor; anxiety; cough; sedation; headache

Occasional: Decreased appetite; sexual dysfunction; dry mouth; constipation; diarrhea; vomiting; dyspepsia; decreased libido; myoclonus; confusion; yawning; blurred vision; taste disturbance; allergic reactions

Rare: Bradycardia; delirium; psychoses; extrapyramidal reactions; platelet dysfunction and bleeding

PERPHENAZINE (*Trilafon*, and others) see Phenothiazines, piperazine

PHENELZINE *(Nardil)*, see MAO inhibitors

PHENOTHIAZINES, ALIPHATIC (chlorpromazine, triflupromazine)

Frequent: Drowsiness; anticholinergic effects;* postural hypotension

Occasional: Extrapyramidal effects; galactorrhea; photosensitivity; menstrual changes; cholestatic jaundice; rashes; skin pigmentation; convulsions; ECG changes; tardive dyskinesia; weight gain

Rare: Lenticular deposits and opacities; blood dyscrasias; gastritis, nausea and vomiting, dizziness and tremulousness following withdrawal of high-dose therapy; disturbed temperature regulation; lupus-like syndrome; neuroleptic malignant syndrome

PHENOTHIAZINES, PIPERAZINE (acetophenazine, fluphenazine, perphenazine, prochlorperazine, trifluoperazine)

Frequent: Extrapyramidal effects
Occasional: Anticholinergic effects;* photosensitivity; galactorrhea; menstrual changes; drowsiness; postural hypotension; anorexia; rash; tardive dyskinesia; weight gain
Rare: Cholestatic jaundice; blood dyscrasias; lenticular deposits and opacities; ECG abnormalities; convulsions; gastritis; neuroleptic malignant syndrome; nausea and vomiting, dizziness and tremulousness following withdrawal of high-dose therapy; disturbed temperature regulation

PHENOTHIAZINES, PIPERIDINE (mesoridazine, thioridazine)

Frequent: Drowsiness; anticholinergic effects;* postural hypotension; weight gain; inhibition of ejaculation
Occasional: Extrapyramidal effects (but less than with aliphatic phenothiazines); menstrual changes; photosensitivity reactions; ECG abnormalities; galactorrhea; tardive dyskinesia
Rare: Pigmentary retinopathy (thioridazine has an 800 mg/day upper limit on recommended dosage because of a high incidence of pigmentary retinopathy); cholestatic jaundice; blood dyscrasias; dystonia; convulsions; rash; gastritis, nausea and vomiting, dizziness and tremulousness following withdrawal of high-dose therapy; disturbed temperature regulation; neuroleptic malignant syndrome; torsades de pointes ventricular arrhythmia with thioridazine

PRAZEPAM, see Benzodiazepines

PROCHLORPERAZINE (*Compazine*, and others) see Phenothiazines, piperazine

PROTRIPTYLINE *(Vivactil)*, see Tricyclic antidepressants

RISPERIDONE *(Risperdal)*

Frequent: Blurred vision; vertigo; postural dizziness; impaired concentration; decreased appetite; sedation; drowsiness; asthenia; headache; nausea
Occasional: Extrapyramidal effects; reflex tachycardia; orthostatic hypotension; problems with erection and ejaculation; elevation of serum prolactin levels; weight gain
Rare: Hypotension; agitation; anxiety; insomnia; neuroleptic malignant syndrome; priapism

SERTRALINE *(Zoloft)*

Frequent: Nausea; headache; diarrhea; insomnia; dry mouth; ejaculatory delay; drowsiness; dizziness; tremor; fatigue; increased sweating
Occasional: Agitation; anxiety; paresthesias; anorexia; palpitations; micturition frequency; hot flushes; asthenia; sexual dysfunction
Rare: Rhinitis; impaired concentration; rash; yawning; myalgia; hypoesthesia; taste disturbances; tinnitus; increased appetite; thirst; extrapyramidal reactions; galactorrhea; platelet dysfunction and bleeding; antidiuresis

TEMAZEPAM (*Restoril*, and others), see Benzodiazepines

THIORIDAZINE (*Mellaril*, and others) see Phenothiazines, piperidine

THIOTHIXENE (*Navane*, and others)
Frequent: Extrapyramidal effects; anticholinergic effects*
Occasional: Galactorrhea; menstrual changes; drowsiness; postural hypotension; anorexia; rash; tardive dyskinesia
Rare: Blood dyscrasias; lenticular deposits and opacities (with long-term high dosage); ECG abnormalities; convulsions; neuroleptic malignant syndrome

TRANYLCYPROMINE *(Parnate)*, see MAO inhibitors

TRAZODONE (*Desyrel*, and others)
Frequent: Drowsiness; headaches; gastrointestinal upset
Occasional: Ventricular arrhythmias; peripheral edema
Rare: Priapism in men; increased libido

TRICYCLIC ANTIDEPRESSANTS (amitriptyline, amoxapine, clomipramine, desipramine, doxepin, imipramine, nortriptyline, protriptyline, trimipramine)
Frequent: Anticholinergic effects;* hypotension (less with nortriptyline); drowsiness; weight gain; tachycardia
Occasional: Mania; psychosis; tremor; first-degree heart block; other ECG abnormalities; rash; sweating; confusion; insomnia; anorgasmia and other sexual disturbances, especially with clomipramine; increase in dental caries; gingivitis; withdrawal symptoms
Rare: Hepatic toxicity; tinnitus; bone marrow depression, including agranulocytosis; seizures, more with clomipramine; peripheral neuropathy; severe cardiovascular effects in patients with cardiac disease; photosensitivity; dysarthria; stuttering; nausea, tremor, and seizures may be more common with clomipramine; tardive dyskinesia and neuroleptic malignant syndrome with amoxapine; renal failure with overdosage of amoxapine

TRIFLUOPERAZINE (*Stelazine*, and others) see Phenothiazines, piperazine

TRIFLUPROMAZINE *(Vesprin)*, see Phenothiazines, aliphatic

TRIMIPRAMINE (*Surmontil*, and others) see Tricyclic antidepressants

VALPROIC ACID (*Depakene*, and others)
Frequent: Nausea
Occasional: Weight gain; hair loss; tremor; rash; insomnia; leukopenia; thrombocytopenia; increased aminotransferase activity
Rare: Fatal hepatic toxicity

VENLAFAXINE *(Effexor)*
Frequent: Nausea; somnolence; dizziness; headache; sweating; anorexia; insomnia; nervousness; anxiety
Occasional: Weight loss; sexual dysfunction; dry mouth; constipation
Rare: Hypotension; hypertension; seizures

---

* Dry mouth, mydriasis, cycloplegia, urinary retention, decreased GI motility, tachycardia, memory impairment and, in high doses, delirium

FOODS INTERACTING WITH MAO INHIBITORS

	Comments
FOOD CONTAINING TYRAMINE	
Avocados	Particularly if overripe[1, 2]
Bananas	Reactions can occur if eaten in large amounts; tyramine levels high in peel.[2, 3]
Bean curd	Fermented bean curd, fermented soya bean, soya bean pastes, soy sauces and miso soup, prepared from fermented bean curd, all contain tyramine in large amounts; miso soup has caused reactions.[4]
Beer and ale	Major domestic bottled brands do not contain appreciable amounts; some imported brands and domestic tap lagers from local breweries have high levels.[5] Nonalcoholic beer may contain tyramine and should be avoided.[6]
Caviar	Safe if vacuum-packed and eaten fresh or refrigerated only briefly[5]
Cheese	Reactions possible with most, except unfermented varieties such as cottage cheese.[5] In others, tyramine concentration is higher near rind and close to fermentation holes.[5]
Figs	Particularly if overripe.[2]
Fish	Safe if fresh; dried products should not be eaten. Caution required in restaurants. Vacuum-packed products are safe if eaten promptly or refrigerated only briefly.[5]
Liver	Safe if very fresh, but rapidly accumulates tyramine; caution required in restaurants.[7]
Milk products	Milk and yogurt appear to be safe.[8]
Protein extracts	See also soups; avoid liquid and powdered protein dietary supplements.[9]
Meat	Safe if known to be fresh; caution required in restaurants.[5, 7]

1. JA Generali et al, Drug Intell Clin Pharm, 15:904, 1981
2. S Udenfriend et al, Arch Biochem Biophys, 85:487, 1959
3. B Blackwell and DC Taylor, Br Med J, 2:381, 1969
4. SK Sung et al, Hum Psychopharmacol, 1:103, 1986; RE Mesmer, JAMA, 258:3515, 1987
5. M Da Prada et al, J Neural Transm, 26 suppl:31, 1988; P Hannah et al, Lancet, 1:879, 1988; SAN Tailor et al, J Clin Psychopharmacol, 14:5, 1994
6. JA Murray et al, Lancet, 1:1167, 1988; R Draper et al, Br Med J, 289:308, 1984; J Thakore et al, Int Clin Psychopharmacol, 7:59, 1992
7. AA Boulton et al, Can Med Assoc J, 102:1394, 1970; ed., Biol Ther Psychiatry, 11:1, 1988
8. D Horwitz et al, JAMA, 188:1108, 1964
9. M Zetin et al, J Clin Psychiatry, 48:499, 1987

	Comments
Sausage	Fermented varieties such as bologna, pepperoni and salami have a high tyramine content.[5]
Shrimp paste	Contains large amounts of tyramine.[4]
Soups	May contain protein extracts and should be avoided.[9]
Soy sauce	Contains large amounts of tyramine; reactions have occurred with teriyaki.[4, 10]
Wines	Generally do not contain tyramine, but many reactions have been reported with Chianti, champagne and other wines.
Yeast extracts	Dietary supplements, e.g. *Marmite*, contain large amounts. Yeast in baked goods, however, is safe.[11]
FOOD NOT CONTAINING TYRAMINE	
Caffeine	A weak pressor agent; large amounts may cause reactions.
Chocolate	Contains phenylethylamine, a pressor agent which can cause reactions in large amounts.[2, 12]
Dietary supplements (weight loss products)	May contain large amounts of cocoa, yeast, and/or yeast extracts.[13]
Fava beans (broad beans, "Italian" green beans)	Contain dopamine, a pressor amine, particularly when overripe.[2]
Ginseng	Some preparations have caused headache, tremulousness and manic-like symptoms.[14]
Liqueurs	Reactions reported with some, e.g. *Chartreuse* and *Drambuie*; cause unknown.
New Zealand prickly spinach	Single case report; patient ate large amounts.[15]
Whiskey	Reactions have occurred; cause unknown.[16]

10. JH Abrams et al, N Engl J Med, 313:52, 1985
11. B Blackwell et al, Lancet, 1:940, 1965
12. DM Krikler and B Lewis, Lancet, 1:1166, 1965
13. RA Sweet et al, J Clin Psychopharmacol, 11:331, 1991
14. BD Jones and AM Runikis, J Clin Psychopharmacol, 7:201, 1987; RI Shader and DJ Greenblatt, J Clin Psychopharmacol, 8:235, 1988
15. A Comfort, Lancet, 2:472, 1981
16. ed., Biol Ther Psychiatry, 11:34, Sept 1988

DRUGS FOR TREATMENT OF PEPTIC ULCERS

Most peptic ulcers not caused by nonsteroidal anti-inflammatory drugs (NSAIDs) are now thought to be associated with infection of the gastric mucosa by the gram-negative bacilli *Helicobacter pylori* (NIH Consensus Development Panel, JAMA, 272:65, 1994). NSAID-related ulcers are usually gastric. *H. pylori* have been associated with both duodenal and gastric ulcers.

ANTIBACTERIAL TREATMENT — Diagnosis – Testing for active *H. pylori* infection currently requires endoscopy and a biopsy of the gastric antrum. Breath tests that require ingestion of radio-labeled urea have been used, but are not yet commercially available. Serologic tests for antibodies to *H. pylori* can also be helpful.

Effectiveness – Eradication of *H. pylori* with various antibacterial combinations has led to rapid healing of active peptic ulcers and low recurrence rates. One 12-month controlled trial in patients with duodenal ulcers and biopsies positive for *H. pylori* found that ulcers recurred in 4 of 50 patients after treatment with an H_2-receptor antagonist plus antibiotics, compared to 42 of 49 given an H_2-receptor antagonist and a placebo (E Hentschel et al, N Engl J Med, 328:308, 1993). Long-term ulcer recurrence rates have also been much lower than usual when *H. pylori* were eradicated (GM Forbes et al, Lancet, 343:258, 1994).

Choice of Drugs – The antibacterial drugs used most often have been bismuth subsalicylate *(Pepto-Bismol)* or subcitrate (not available in the USA), tetracycline hydrochloride (*Achromycin V*, and others), metronidazole (*Flagyl*, and others), amoxicillin (*Amoxil*, and others), and clarithromycin *(Biaxin)*, usually two or three together with an antisecretory drug. Concurrent use of bismuth subsalicylate, 2 tablets q.i.d., tetracycline 500 mg q.i.d., and metronidazole 250 mg t.i.d. for two weeks, usually with an H_2-blocker such as ranitidine *(Zantac)*, has been considered the treatment of choice, but drug toxicity and increasing resistance to metronidazole have caused some concern (European Study Group, Eur J Clin Microbiol Infect Dis, 11:777, 1992). One controlled trial found that concurrent use of amoxicillin, 500 mg q.i.d., with omeprazole, 20 mg b.i.d. for two weeks was about as effective as bismuth subsalicylate, tetracycline, metronidazole and ranitidine, with a lower incidence of adverse effects (J Labenz et al, Gut, 34:1167, 1993). Use of omeprazole with clarithromycin or with bismuth, tetracycline and metronidazole has also been effective (RPH Logan et al, Gut, 35:323, 1994; W de Boer et al, Lancet, 345:817, 1995).

Adverse Effects – Bismuth subsalicylate temporarily turns the tongue and stool black and can cause mild tinnitus. Tetracycline and metronidazole often cause gastrointestinal and other toxicity that may prevent completion of treatment. Amoxicillin is generally well tolerated.

H_2-RECEPTOR ANTAGONISTS — H_2-receptor antagonists inhibit the action of histamine at the histamine H_2-receptor of the parietal cell, decreasing both basal and food-stimulated acid secretion. The four drugs in this class marketed in the USA for treatment of peptic ulcers are all about equally effective. Once-daily bedtime doses have been as effective as more frequent doses, at least for patients with uncomplicated duodenal ulcers. Giving half the acute treatment dose for long-term maintenance has been effective in decreasing the incidence of relapse, particularly in patients who have had bleeding or other complications (DM Jensen et al, N Engl J Med, 330:382, 1994).

Adverse Effects – Severe adverse effects are uncommon with H_2-receptor blockers, but headache, lethargy, confusion, depression and hallucinations can occur. Rarely, these agents have been associated with hepatitis, hematologic toxicity or dystonia. Cimetidine, in particular, may act as an anti-androgen and cause reversible impotence and gynecomastia.

Drug Interactions – Cimetidine inhibits the activity of hepatic cytochrome P-450 enzymes and may interfere with the hepatic metabolism of other drugs. Clinically significant effects have occurred when cimetidine was used with P-450-metabolized drugs with a narrow therapeutic-to-toxic ratio, such as theophylline, warfarin (*Coumadin*, and others), phenytoin (*Dilantin*, and others) or lidocaine (*Xylocaine*, and others) (*Medical Letter Handbook of Adverse Drug Interactions*, 1995, page 55). Ranitidine, famotidine and nizatidine are less likely to interact with other drugs.

PROTON PUMP INHIBITORS — Omeprazole (*Prilosec* – Medical Letter, 32:19, 1990) binds to the proton pump of the parietal cell, inhibiting secretion of hydrogen ions into the gastric lumen. In doses of 20 to 40 mg/day, it inhibits more than 90% of 24-hour acid secretion, compared with 50% to 80% with standard doses of H_2-antagonists. With higher doses, acid inhibition is nearly complete. The drug has a short serum half-life, but one dose acts for more than 24 hours. Omeprazole relieves pain and heals peptic ulcers more rapidly than H_2-antagonists (P Maton, N Engl J Med, 324:965, 1990). Lansoprazole (*Prevacid* – TAP), a second proton pump inhibitor, was approved for marketing by the US Food and Drug Administration in May, 1995.

Adverse Effects – Omeprazole usually causes few adverse effects. Painful nocturnal erections and gynecomastia have occurred rarely (JP Dutertre et al, Lancet, 338:1022, 1991; C Convens et al, Lancet, 338:1153, 1991). Subacute myopathy, arthralgias, severe rashes, and acute interstitial nephritis have been reported (FJ Garrote et al, Lancet, 340:672, 1992; NH Cox, Lancet, 340:857, 1992; PB Christensen et al, Lancet, 341:55, 1993; M Beutler et al, BMJ, 309:1620, 1994).

Drug Interactions – Omeprazole inhibits the activity of some hepatic P-450 enzymes, decreasing the clearance of diazepam (*Valium*, and others), warfarin, and phenytoin. It may also increase absorption of digoxin and decrease the effectiveness of prednisone.

SUCRALFATE — An aluminum hydroxide complex of sucrose, sucralfate (*Carafate* – Medical Letter, 26:43, 1984) has been effective for acute treatment of peptic ulcers and for prevention of relapse. Its mechanism of action is not clear, but it may protect the ulcer from exposure to acid. Multiple daily doses are required, and pain relief is not as effective as with omeprazole or an H_2-blocker. Sucralfate can prevent stress ulcer in mechanically ventilated patients, resulting in less late-onset pneumonia than occurs after prophylactic use of ranitidine or antacids (G Prod'hom et al, Ann Intern Med, 120:653, 1994).

Adverse Effects — Only a small amount of sucralfate is absorbed from the gastrointestinal tract, and the drug has no known serious adverse effects. Constipation can occur. Plasma and urinary levels of aluminum may increase and in patients with chronic renal failure, aluminum toxicity might develop (DJ Sherrard, N Engl J Med, 324:558, 1991). Sucralfate decreases absorption of ketoconazole *(Nizoral)*, fluoroquinolone antibiotics, and other drugs; concurrent medications should be taken at least two hours before sucralfate.

MISOPROSTOL — Misoprostol (*Cytotec* – Medical Letter, 31:21, 1989), a prostaglandin analog, is less effective than an H_2-blocker for acute treatment of peptic ulcers, but can prevent gastric ulcers in patients on chronic NSAID therapy. Some clinicians prescribe misoprostol for patients taking NSAIDs who have a high risk of NSAID-associated complications, such as the elderly, those with multiple medical problems and patients with previous ulcer complications. Dose-related diarrhea is the most common adverse effect, but severe nausea can also occur, especially with the 200 µg dose; 100 µg is better tolerated and almost as effective. Like other prostaglandins, misoprostol is an abortifacient and is contraindicated for use during pregnancy.

ANTACIDS — Aluminum- and magnesium-containing antacids can be effective in promoting healing of duodenal ulcers. The effectiveness of antacids for maintenance to prevent relapse or for treatment of acute gastric ulcer is less well established.

CONCLUSION — When patients with active peptic ulcers not related to NSAIDs are infected with *Helicobacter pylori*, use of antibacterial drugs for two weeks in addition to an H_2-receptor antagonist or omeprazole can decrease the incidence of recurrence.

SOME DRUGS FOR TREATMENT OF PEPTIC ULCERS

Drug	Dosage	Wholesale cost[1]
Antibacterials		
Bismuth subsalicylate – *Pepto Bismol* (Procter & Gamble)	2 tablets qid	$ 10.86
Tetracycline	500 mg qid	
average generic price		5.36
Sumycin (Apothecon)		5.87
Metronidazole	250 mg tid	
average generic price		6.45
Flagyl (Searle)		54.84
Amoxicillin	500 mg qid	
average generic price		18.82
Amoxil (SK Beecham)		22.62
Clarithromycin – *Biaxin* (Abbott)	500 mg tid	124.81
H_2-receptor antagonists		
Cimetidine – average generic price	400 mg bid	$ 78.50
Tagamet (SK Beecham)		92.60
Famotidine – *Pepcid* (Merck)	20 mg bid	92.48
Nizatidine – *Axid* (Lilly)	150 mg bid	92.31
Ranitidine – *Zantac* (Glaxo)	150 mg bid	95.66
Omeprazole – *Prilosec* (Merck)	20 mg once[2]	108.90
Sucralfate – *Carafate* (Marion Merrell Dow)	1 gram qid	88.43
Misoprostol[3] – *Cytotec* (Searle)	200 µg qid	84.76
Magnesium hydroxide/aluminum hydroxide/simethicone antacids		
Maalox Extra Strength Antacid (Rhône-Poulenc Rorer)	2 tablets qid	20.38
Mylanta Double Strength (Johnson & Johnson)	2 tablets qid	19.12

1. Cost to the pharmacist for 14 days' treatment with antibacterials and 30 days' treatment with other drugs, based on wholesale price (AWP) listings in *Drug Topics Red Book* 1995 and May *Update*.
2. For use with amoxicillin to eradicate *H. pylori*, dosage is 20 mg b.i.d.
3. FDA-approved only for treatment of NSAID-associated gastric ulcers.